I0823061

How to Deal with Your (   )
So Your Kids Don't Have To*

*as much

How to Deal with Your ( ) So Your Kids Don't Have To*

AN ENCYCLOPEDIA FOR DITCHING YOUR EMOTIONAL BAGGAGE

ELI HARWOOD, MA, LPC

*as much

Printed in China

SASQUATCH BOOKS with colophon is a registered trademark
of Blue Star Press, LLC

10 9 8 7 6 5 4 3 2 1

The authorized representative in the EU for product safety and compliance is Authorised Rep Compliance Ltd., Ground Floor, 71 Lower Baggot Street, Dublin D02 P593, Ireland. www.arccompliance.com

Editor: Jill Saginario | Production editor: Peggy Gannon
Inclusivity editor: Diana Cherry | Designer: Anna Goldstein
Cover art: Maricor/Maricar

Library of Congress Cataloging-in-Publication Data is available.

ISBN: 978-1-63217-596-0

Sasquatch Books | 1325 Fourth Avenue, Suite 1025 | Seattle, WA 98101

SasquatchBooks.com

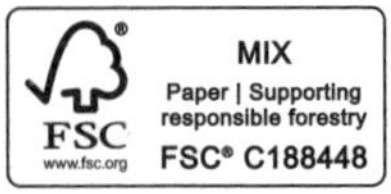

This book is dedicated to my mom, who courageously lit a path of healing for me to follow and then continued to cheer me on even when that path meant I needed to illuminate and process pain from my childhood. And to my brother, who has been blazing this trail at warp speed. I am so amazed by you and so thankful that you are with me on this mission.

Contents

Introduction

I know very few parents who intentionally choose to pass on problematic habits, immature emotional patterns, or generational trauma to their children. The overwhelming majority of us truly want the best for our kids and feel sick to our stomachs at the thought of being a source of disconnection, struggle, or trauma in their lives. And since you chose to pick up this book, I'm going to assume that's also true for you.

Like me you want your children to experience a secure childhood and a long-term positive relationship with you. You want to be able to give your children a healthier developmental experience than you had when you were growing up. Even if what you had was pretty darn good. And if your children are already grown, then you want to be able to mend the past and improve your relationship with them moving forward.

We are in the same club! We're not the *perfect parent* club or the *parents who always know exactly what to do* club; we're the *parents who are willing to deal with our sh*t because we're passionate about having positive relationships with our children* club. (Let me know if you can think of something catchier, obviously.)

I wrote this book for us because I want us to have the maps, tools, and resources we need to avoid the pain of accidentally continuing (or creating) insecure, disconnected, or painful dynamics in our relationships with our offspring, whether they are two or fifty-two.

It's a quest my mom started in my family, and it's one that my siblings and I are working to continue. Thankfully it's a quest that has been journeyed by many courageous parents, and it has been validated as a worthy cause in the rich body of research on the parent-child relationship over the past century, or close to it.

It's not an easy quest, but that's part of what makes it so profoundly impactful. The discomfort and challenges we encounter on this journey to becoming more emotionally reliable for our children are absolutely worth the cost. As we learn and grow, we not only develop better relationships with our children but also cultivate more peace, self-acceptance, and clarity on what matters in our lives.

The Five Gifts of a Secure Parent

Since developing secure relationships with our children is the most powerful parenting flex we have, let's quickly review the five core experiences that our children require to feel truly secure in their relationships with us.

1. **The gift of feeling that we can handle their emotions**
   "My parent cares about what I feel and knows how to support me."

2. **The gift of feeling that we understand their perspectives**
   "My parent listens to me and works to truly understand me."

3. **The gift of feeling that we want them close to us**
   "My parent lights up when I enter the room. They love being around me."

4. **The gift of feeling that we show up for them in important moments**
   "My parent shows up for me when I'm struggling and when I'm celebrating."

5. **The gift of feeling that we accept them for their full, authentic selves**
   "My parent is proud of every part of me."

The Sh*t That Gets in the Way of Secure

Now that we have some clear goals of what we want to be able to offer our children, let's get to the core reason for this particular book's existence: the five gifts of a secure parent are far easier said than done! To give our children those experiences, we have to be *relatively emotionally mature*. We must know how to handle the incredibly complex landscape of human emotion without getting stuck in habits and reactions that lead to disconnection and alienation from our kids.

We don't have to be perfectly emotionally regulated all the time, that would make us robots. But there are certain habitual pitfalls that we should try to avoid and emotional skills we need to develop in order to cultivate the trust and emotional closeness our children need from us.

Let's think about our relationship with our children as a video game. We'll call it *Super Mario Parents*. Mostly because *Super Mario Brothers* was one of two video games I played growing up (the other one being *The Oregon Trail*, which always ended with me dying of dysentery).

The goal of our *Super Mario Parents* game is to create and retain a positive and close relationship with our children throughout each new level (age/stage).

As we walk/run/jump through each level, we encounter obstacles that can block us from winning the game. In *Super Mario Parents* the goal of the game is to protect our relationship with our children.

And just like any game worth playing, there are weird evil mushroom dudes trying to take us down. Things like unresolved trauma, perfectionism, and control habits. These "goombas" can really mess things up for us and our kids and prevent us from giving them the five gifts they need from us (page x).

We are most effective in our human parenting quest when we are able to acknowledge our growth areas (our sh*t) with both self-compassion *and* determination to grow.

The Process of Dealing with Our Sh*t

I highly doubt that you will relate to every topic in this book. Especially because we all hold unique experiences and cultural backgrounds that influence our particular growth needs. No need to read it all at once or in any particular order. Use it as a reference guide to help you answer the questions, "How is my sh*t affecting my relationship with kids?" And "What can I be doing to grow more emotionally connected and sturdy?"

I hope that reading this book will give you:

1. A shower of ah-ha moments! *"I recognize this negative attribute or habit in myself."*
2. Motivation to make changes! *"I see how this could affect my children and why they deserve my efforts to address this thing."*

3. Increased compassion toward yourself! *"I also see why I've handled this issue the way I have up until now, and I know it doesn't mean I'm a bad parent."*
4. Efforts toward growth! *"I'm going to take the steps necessary to change the impact this issue has on me and my children."*

You'll also discover that some of these struggles overlap—a bit like baggage sets. If you struggle with managing anger (page 9), you may also struggle with a numbing habit (page 208). If you struggle with a people-pleasing habit (page 224), you may also struggle with a perfectionism habit (page 231). This is 100 percent normal. I'm working through a solid handful of these issues myself ("stress-mess" is my middle name!), and I know and love and respect people navigating things in every single category here.

Each topic is organized around these nuggets:

1. A description of the issue
2. A description of how the issue could negatively affect our children
3. Practical things we can do to mature and grow around the issue
4. Compassionate self-talk scripts: examples of things we can say to *ourselves* around the topic to encourage us to offer compassion to ourselves as we work on these issues
5. Further reading recommendations* to help us dig deeper into our understanding of the topic

---

*Note that I do not agree with every single thing in all the recommended books and resources listed, and you don't need to either. Find the resources that feel helpful to you, take the parts that resonate for your journey, and ignore the rest! We don't need to align on *everything* to be able to support each other in *some things.*

Plus:

- **Trusty Tidbits:** snack-sized insights and advice sprinkled throughout to help us become the trustworthy parents we want to be
- **Stop Signs:** alerts to habits or emotional states that deserve *urgent* support (If you resonate with a Stop Sign, please stop reading and reach out to someone you trust, or to a community resource, and ask for support with the issue that you recognized in yourself.)

Most important of all, I hope we can all hold onto the truth that the goombas on our path are not issues that *bad* parents struggle with, they're issues that *human* parents struggle with.

This Won't Be a Walk in the Park, but . . .

I will do my best to keep you feeling engaged, and I will definitely make a joke or two. But overall I'm guessing this book is going to feel less like a pedicure and more like getting a toenail or two surgically removed. (And as someone who is personally down one toenail, I can tell you that it's not the worst medical procedure to go through, but it sure ain't fun. *Rest in peace, big toenail from my right foot.*)

Growth is rarely a walk in the park. In my almost two decades as a therapist, I don't think anyone has ever left my office after facing a growth moment and said, "That was fun! I wish I could do this every day!"

But just because it's work and not necessarily fun doesn't mean it won't come with a tremendous amount of fulfillment and relief. It took me ten years to finally decide to remove my toenail. It had been unruly and mean to my foot for a long time, growing in the wrong direction and wreaking havoc on my ability to wear pointy-toed shoes. It was uncomfortable (and a bit expensive) to say adieu to my malfunctioning nail, but the relief I've felt since I finally let it go has been well worth the pain it took to remove it.

Just like hiking up a mountain, this book will involve using your muscles, feeling tired, wanting to turn back at times, and acquiring a few blisters. *But*, and this is a *big* "but," (*big butt*—haha! Sorry—I spend a ton of time with my twin five-year-olds) *the view from the top is exquisite.*

Remember the gift of perspective can only come as a result of having walked up a hill. I hope that as you work through the topics in this book, you'll find yourself surrounded by beautiful views. Even if that means you lose a toenail in the process.

Heroes Have Allies

You might be able to battle a few of these topics on your own, but most of them will be far easier to handle with help. I can say with confidence that there is no wiser choice in life than the decision to seek the support of others. For so many of us carrying generational trauma, asking for help feels like failure. But in reality it is often one of our greatest achievements.

Emotional growth, healing, and change are *team sports.*

Confide in sweethearts, friends, and trusted mentors, or find a therapist or support group that you genuinely feel connected to. (For more specifics on how to find a good therapist, check the Think of Finding a Therapist as a Dating Process section on page 267.)

Warning: Awards, Acknowledgments, and Gratitude Are Not Guaranteed

Unlike public feats of heroism, our journeys to heal generational patterns are private and lack the expected glory that we deserve for doing something heroic.

When we break cycles on behalf of our children, we also create a reality in which they cannot understand what we've done for them.

If we can ensure that our children have enough food to eat, they won't understand the pains of starvation that we protect them from. Without the ache of a chronically empty belly, our children can't comprehend what a privilege it is to complain about the food on their plates instead of worrying that their plates are empty.

That's what generational progress looks like. We've changed the game. The fact that their understanding of "suffering" is different from ours also means their feelings of gratitude will be different. If our children are "ungrateful" to us for preventing them from experiencing so many painful realities, it means we've successfully separated them from those things.

Even though our children may not be handing us parent of the year awards, that doesn't mean we won't feel the benefits of this work. We will be rewarded with close and authentic relationships with our children. We can savor the gift of knowing that our children intuitively trust that we're people they can rely on when life gets crusty, musty, and tender.

And we can always celebrate *ourselves*. I feel very proud of myself when I deal with one of these issues in my life. I take time to reflect on what I've done and let it seep into my identity and self-assurance. I am a mama on a mission, determined to give my kids a parent who is as emotionally healthy as possible. Sometimes just telling myself I am doing a good job is enough. Other days I give myself a nap or a cookie.

If you need more acknowledgment, celebration, or reward during this journey, invite friends to celebrate you. Just don't invite your kids. It's not their responsibility, and since they don't understand the pain that you protected them from, they can't possibly give you the type of gratitude you are craving and deserve.

A Word on Obstacle Courses

"Wanna fly, you got to give up
the shit that weighs you down."
—**TONI MORRISON**, *Song of Solomon*

None of us are playing the same version of *Super Mario Parents*. It's *so* important to remember this as we seek to work on ourselves and heal. We're not all given the same number of coins or extra lives to help us survive obstacles along our way. And we aren't facing the same volume of goombas in our way.

As a heterosexual American woman with European ancestry, a supportive partner, a steady job, and legal status in my country of residence, I have a ton of advantages on my cycle-breaking journey.

But we are not all equally supported and accepted by society.

- Some of us have obstacles of significant wreckage from childhood trauma.
- Some of us have obstacles of neurodivergence, either our own or our children's.
- Some of us have obstacles of social/identity oppression and trauma.
- Some of us have obstacles of mental health struggles.
- Some of us have the obstacle of parenting without a partner or family support.
- Some of us have the obstacle of an abusive relationship.
- Some of us have the obstacle of financial insecurity.
- Some of us have the obstacle of war and rampant violence in our communities.

It is important that we do the best we can with what we have and remember that we're all playing different versions of the game.

I: The Feelings

One of the most important things we do for our children is learn how to maturely handle the tricky feelings that inevitably arise inside us as parents. For us to give them the first gift of a secure parent, *to feel that we can handle what they feel*, we have to be able to respond effectively in emotional moments.

Of course this is no small feat.

Learning how to cope with our feelings while our children are bubbling over with emotions *at the same time* is like trying to learn addition and subtraction in the middle of an algebra class. Even as a trained professional at handling feelings, I'm still regularly blind-sided by the intense onslaught of emotions that comes with being a parent.

Before we consider specific feeling states, let's assess how we generally relate to our emotions.

Avoidant Attachment

If: Feelings Make You Want to Flee

You Might Have: An Avoidant Emotional Pattern (colloquially known as an avoidant attachment style)

Imagine that you grew up in a home where no one ever talked about football. Your family had a thing against football, and your parents got annoyed when a neighbor or a teacher had the audacity to acknowledge the sport. You had a vague idea of what football was, but you knew nothing about the rules of the game, how to score, how to defend, or even what gear to wear. You've always endeavored to stay away from football because you've been taught that it's bad, and you don't really want to find out why.

Now imagine that one day you're told that you've been put in charge of a football team. Your job is to teach your team how to be successful on the field. Without a clue of how to play yourself. (This would be me, the only things I know about football I learned watching *Friday Night Lights!* Go Tim Riggins!)

Unfortunately for so many parents this is the reality we face when we first meet our children. We are given the task of helping our children learn to navigate their feelings, when our only training has been to *avoid feelings altogether.*

This looks like:

- Ignoring, punishing, or distracting our children when they melt down
- Apologizing, coughing it away, distracting ourselves, or leaving the room when *we* feel emotional

- Believing that emotions are weak, useless, or burdensome to others
- Dismissing our children's painful emotions by telling them they are "fine"
- Getting frustrated or despondent when we or our children are emotional
- Using a small vocabulary of words to describe our emotions or to help our children describe theirs (If the only feeling words you use to describe your inner states are "fine," "okay," or "great," you probably need some more words to share your emotions with the people you love.)

Our children are wired to seek us out as a safe haven during emotional storms. If we avoid their feelings or respond dismissively when they're upset, they'll quickly learn to stop coming to us in their tender moments. And if they don't have an emotionally available substitute adult, they will also learn to avoid their feelings as their primary coping pattern.

Remember this: teaching a child to ignore their emotions is not teaching them how to *calm down*, it's teaching them how to *shut down*. Calm, a.k.a. regulated, is a state we experience when we sense that our feelings are understood and accepted and that we don't have to handle them in isolation.

Teaching our children that it is okay to feel and that we will be there to support them is the path toward helping them develop confidence, empathy, and resilience. Even when it's incredibly inconvenient, as it so often is.

Tips for avoiding avoidance (see what I did there?):

1 Increase the amount of time you allow yourself to feel your feelings.

2. Spend more time checking in with your own body sensations throughout the day and labeling them with feeling words.
3. Communicate actively with your children that you are working on becoming more comfortable with feelings and emotions.
4. Move toward your children when they are emotional so they can sense that you care and want to be near them even when they are "full of feels."

Anxious Attachment

If: You Can't Stop the Feelings

You Might Have: A Preoccupied Emotional Pattern (colloquially known as an anxious attachment style)

For others of us, feeling our feelings is our game. We bathe in feelings. We obsess about feelings. We feel feelings about our feelings until other feelings take over. This emotional pattern is also a coping mechanism. Obsessing about what we feel and what our children feel is an attempt to stay alert to changes in emotions that could lead to a loss of connection. It's how we handle our deep-seated fear of abandonment.

An obsession with emotions makes us preoccupied with them and distracts us from a secure experience. This pattern keeps us anxious and oversensitive to our children's emotions.

This looks like:

- Scanning our children constantly for their feeling states
- Catastrophizing the presence of feelings
- Worrying that we're failing as parents if our children are upset
- Asking about feelings every other minute "just to make sure"
- Feeling calm only when our children feel calm, and feeling lost and upset when they feel lost and upset

This approach to feelings is also problematic for our relationships with our children, as it leads us to hover and to cultivate an intrusive vibe in response to their emotional states. If Goldilocks had something to say here about preoccupied porridge, it would be that it's too hot! (The avoidant porridge would be too cold.)

While our children need us to notice and feel emotions, they also need us to be capable of *tolerating* and *managing* them. We want to show our children that we can have our feelings without our feelings controlling us.

Tips for calming a preoccupied porridge:

1. Limit questioning your children about feelings and emotions to once or twice a day.
2. Write yourself a note on your mirror that says, "It is not my job to prevent my children from feeling emotional discomfort or pain; it's my job to prevent them from feeling alone in their pain."
3. Start and end your day with a short relaxation exercise to calm your nervous system.
4. Use phrases like *"we will figure this out"* and *"I'm here, I got you"* to remind yourself and your children that you can handle what they feel.

Disorganized Attachment

If: Feelings Feel Dangerous

You Might Have: A Disorganized Emotional Pattern (colloquially known as a disorganized attachment style)

When feelings (especially the tender and challenging ones) feel scary or deeply unsettling, it's usually due to a history with caregivers or partners who frightened us. They held abusive mindsets or had severe mental illnesses or drug addictions that caused them to act in erratic and frightening ways when we were emotional. The internal wires for *"I am feeling something"* became linked with the wires for *"Something really bad is about to happen,"* activating our threat response systems when emotions were present.

This is especially true if we were punished for having feelings. (I'm thinking about a dear client who was locked in a closet as a child for crying at bedtime; he wasn't allowed to leave the dark, lonely closet until he stopped crying.) In these cases our relationships to feelings are deeply influenced by our traumatic experiences.

These traumatic experiences are embedded in our nervous systems and make it hard for us to feel safe, even when the feelings are coming from our small children who hold no real power over us and need our help to learn how to regulate their emotions.

This looks like:

- Getting angry or enraged at our children when they are tender or sad
- Assuming that our children are trying to gain power over us or hurt us when they're struggling emotionally or behaviorally
- Experiencing trauma reactions, including fight, flight, freeze, faint, or fawn, when our children are feeling frustrated or angry
- Shutting down and going numb when our children are upset
- Feeling justified in calling our children names or shaming them when they are in a state of distress

Tips for organizing our responses to feelings:

1 Seek out trauma focused therapy to help you separate past trauma from present needs.
2 Set a daily alarm on your phone that says, "My children are not giving me a hard time, they are having a hard time."
3 Be as compassionate toward your own emotional states as you can. The more you treat your tender emotional states with compassion, the easier it will be to do the same for your kids.

Secure Attachment

If: Feelings Feel Important and Manageable

You Might Have: A Secure Emotional Pattern (colloquially known as a secure attachment style)

This is what I want for all of us. To be able to notice what we feel, uncover whatever needs are cradled within those feelings, and then respond effectively to those needs.

When we have a secure pattern with emotions, we understand that *feelings are helpers.*

Our feelings can inform us about what is happening at any moment (or what happened in a past moment that's being triggered in a present moment) and can offer us guidance on how to navigate the moment successfully. While our emotions can occasionally get unruly (particularly when we've been up all night), they're ultimately here *for* us. If we work *with* them instead of trying to shut them down or blow them up, our feelings will bolster our well-being.

This looks like:

- Offering compassion when our children feel tender
- Validating our children when they feel angry or upset
- Guiding our children in effective coping strategies that help them move through their emotions instead of shutting them down
- Apologizing and repairing when we're not able to offer care or concern immediately
- Modeling acknowledgment of feelings within ourselves
- Recognizing when our present feelings are actually about past experiences
- Taking the time to regulate our bodies when our feelings are flooding us or making it hard for us to make kind and calm choices

How to Deal with Feeling Angry

"Focused with precision, anger can become a powerful source of energy serving progress and change."

—**AUDRE LORDE**, *The Uses of Anger: Women Responding to Racism*

Having angry feelings does not make us bad parents, and our children aren't being bad when they're feeling angry. Anger is a core human emotion, albeit a tricky one to learn how to tolerate and manage.

How we feel about anger depends on the cultures we grew up in and the identities we held within them. For example, as a girl growing up I intuitively learned that anger was "unbecoming" for my gender. If I showed any anger, I could easily be labeled as "difficult" or worse. Whereas if the boys around me showed anger, they were far less likely to be negatively labeled for having it. This taught me to turn my anger inward, seeing it as a liability. It's taken me many years in therapy to learn to trust my anger and to see it as an important piece of information in my body.

Whatever cultural messages we've absorbed about anger, we need to identify and evaluate them so we can choose which messages are helpful, and which messages need to be flushed down the toilet.

Regardless of the different attitudes we learned about anger growing up, our children need us to develop a positive relationship with it now so that we can be an example and resource for them when they are feeling angry.

"But lady," you say, "anger is destructive and dangerous—I've seen it first-hand!" You're not wrong. Anger *can be* incredibly detrimental, but only when it isn't acting alone. Anger gets out of control when it is caught up with shady influences such as *abusive beliefs, toxic entitlement*, or *explosive expressions or behaviors.*

But when anger is not under the influence of those other destructive characters, it's simply a flashlight that illuminates needs that require our attention. If we're feeling desperate or are being harassed, mistreated, neglected, or misunderstood—or we're watching this happen to someone we care about:

Anger's job is to motivate us to take action to care for ourselves and others when something important has gone awry. Anger is a helper.

If we put in the work to understand our angry feelings and manage our responses to them, we can teach our children to do the same.

I have worked very hard to befriend my anger and see "her" as an ally in my journey to stay alive and to have healthy relationships. Now when she knocks on my door, I greet her with curiosity, knowing that she always has something to share with me about what I am needing.

She might knock when my kids ruin something I care about. She knocked very clearly one day when I took a three-minute potty break and returned to our living room to discover that my brand-spanking-new couch had been covered in a red Sharpie abstract art piece that could only be titled *The Eighteen-Month-Old Twins Somehow Got Marker Contraband.*

I dramatically snatched the Sharpies off the couch and told my twins, "Mommy is mad and needs some space to let out her anger," then I ran out to the porch to have a good old-fashioned temper tantrum. My anger was directing me to process a loss I had to face—the loss of the delusion that I could buy a new couch and keep it clean with small rugrats still at large in my family.

After I stomped and grunted enough to get some of my anger out, I googled all the possible ways to remove Sharpie from a leather couch. I was then able to gain some perspective and even laugh a little. This is why we can't have nice things. Or Sharpies.

Anger also shows up in far more serious situations, such as when someone is being mistreated or an injustice is playing out on an individual or group scale. Anger motivates us to process violations and unfair circumstances. In its pure form it guides us to take action by listening, witnessing, and offering whatever support we can.

How Does Our Anger Affect Our Children?

As long as our anger is managed and handled maturely, it acts as a model for our children. But alas many of us did not have those examples in our own childhoods. Here are some different unhealthy generational anger goombas that can get in the way of us offering our children what they need from us.

"I Am Never Angry"

If we ignore, deny, or bury our angry feelings, we are also looking away from what the anger is trying to help us address. And if we never allow ourselves to acknowledge and feel our anger, we can't help our children with theirs. Suppressing and ignoring anger is not the same as having a healthy relationship with it.

Examples of anger suppression in parenting:

- Leaving the room immediately when we're angry, or our children are angry, and waiting until the feelings subside without acknowledging or addressing the anger (avoidance)
- Pretending that we're not angry and changing focus away from our anger to hide it from our children (denial)
- Denying that we're angry when our children ask or point it out to us (gaslighting)
- Focusing attention on "positive things" when we are faced with angry feelings (toxic positivity)

If we're never able to feel our anger, it will compromise our ability to offer our children gift #1, to show them we can handle their emotions. If they sense that we can't manage our own anger, they will not trust us to truly empathize with theirs.

It can also compromise gift #4, compromising our ability to show up for them when they are experiencing violations or struggles that involve anger.

Lastly it can compromise our ability to give them gift #5, for them to feel that we accept and celebrate them for their full, authentic selves. This is especially true for those children who have fire inside their bones around injustice. If we try to suppress their anger like we have our own, it might put out their light or teach them to hide it from us.

"I Lose Control When I Feel Angry"

Anger can also become a problem in our lives and our children's lives if we don't know how to manage our responses to it. If we react and escalate when we're angry, our children will probably feel afraid of us. And if that's the case, they have only two options in response—to hide from us or to escalate their own anger to battle us.

Examples of out-of-control anger in parenting:

- Reacting with a harsh voice and angry facial expression when our children make mistakes (we all do this from time to time—it is a problem if we do it often and without repair and accountability after)
- Justifying intimidating behavior toward our children when they feel angry or defiant in some way toward us
- Fixating on how we feel the world has wronged us as our primary view of our story
- Blowing up at our children, or anyone else in our lives, in front of our children when we feel angry
- Giving our children, or other people, the silent treatment or "stonewalling" them when we feel angry
- Raging at other drivers on the road when they aren't behaving how we want them to
- Using denigrating terms or intimidating postures with strangers in real life or with people on the internet or television

It is *never* okay to turn our anger into physical harm toward our children. Nor is it okay to turn our anger into insults or threats directed at our children. (If you do this, see the Stop Sign on page 15.) Our children have a right to emotional and physical safety, and it is our job to do whatever it takes to keep our children safe, even when we are full of outrage about their behavior or dysregulation.

If our anger is out of control, it prevents our children from receiving gift #1, to feel that we can handle their emotions, because it shows them that we cannot even handle our own.

It also gets in the way of gift #2, to feel that we care about their perspectives, because our anger leads them to hide their feelings and needs out of fear that they'll trigger an eruption in us. As well as messing up #4, to feel that we show up for them in important moments, because our out-of-control anger becomes a source of fear for them, and we can't help them if we are the cause of their distress.

"I Feel Angry All the Time"

When we feel angry all the time, our children come to see us as angry people. They'll most likely avoid any opportunities for closeness with us because they don't want to be near the tension that our presence brings into the room.

Being chronically angry is always an indicator that something is significantly awry in our life or within ourselves.

We might have unresolved trauma (page 142) that puts us on edge and leaves us reactive, exhausted, and angry.

We might be stuck in a situation that leaves us feeling unsafe and constantly on guard (such as abuse).

We might have problematic beliefs and expectations of ourselves or others that trigger constant anger.

We might have unaddressed mental health needs.

When we're angry all the time, it gets in the way of all five gifts of a secure parent (page x). We cannot offer our children regulation, support, delight, understanding, or full permission to be themselves with us if we're constantly embroiled in an anger cloud. Our energy becomes repellent to their nervous systems. If we want to give them those five gifts, we have to figure out how to live outside of an angry emotional state.

STOP

If you have ever resorted to physically harming your child (or are feeling the urge to) in the heat of an angry moment, it's a strong indicator that you're drowning in trauma and dysregulation, and you need some extra care and support to stop a destructive train.

I don't want you to feel like I'm bossing you around, but I know that when I'm in a potentially desperate place, it can be comforting to receive clear, step-by-step guidance.

Please be kind to yourself. This is not a sign that you're a monster; it's a sign that you're struggling.

Immediately call someone you trust and ask them to help you in whatever way relieves some of the present desperation you're feeling.

Reach out to the resources trained to help, such as:

a. US-based mental health resources for parents: Mental Health America (MHANational.org) | Prevent Child Abuse America (PreventChildAbuse.org)
b. Parent-Child Interaction Therapy, which has been shown to prevent child maltreatment by addressing behavioral concerns in children aged two to seven: PCIT International (PCIT.org)
c. International resources for parents: Global Initiative to Support Parents (Support-Parents.org) | UNICEF Parenting (UNICEF.org/parenting)

Trusty Tidbit

TIPS FOR EFFECTIVE APOLOGIES

1 Make Apologizing a Relational Rhythm

Apologizing to our kids is a powerful way to earn trust. It shows our children that we care more about our relationship with them than we do about having control over them. It also normalizes being human and making mistakes from time to time (or every day if you're like me).

2 Don't Over-Apologize

If we apologize for every breath we take or every time our children are remotely uncomfortable, it can dilute the effectiveness of an apology. Over-apologizing is a trauma response, and it communicates to our children that we feel insecure about our place in the world. This makes it harder for them to trust that we can be relied on.

3 Forgive Yourself Before You Apologize

We must always forgive ourselves before apologizing to our children. Why? Because we will be looking for them to forgive us instead of helping them to feel seen, validated, and supported in connection to whatever we did or didn't do.

And when we respond to ourselves compassionately after messing up with our kids, it helps them learn to respond compassionately to their own mistakes.

4 Learn from Your Mistakes

When we say we're sorry but make no efforts to change or learn from the pain we caused someone else, our apologies lose significant luster. The most powerful apologies are followed up by genuine change and ongoing awareness.

Let's Grow!

Dealing with angry feelings is a bit like Goldilocks and her process of finding the right porridge temperature. We don't want to shove our anger away so far that we're disconnected from the wisdom it brings us (toooooo cold). We also don't want to blow it all around the room and unleash emotional or physical fists anytime we feel angry (toooooo hot). We want to show our children how to notice, understand, and respond to anger in ways that lead to greater self and community care (juuuust right).

Here are the growth steps required to learn how to manage anger:

Acknowledge Angry Feelings

The first step to managing our anger is to simply (and compassionately) acknowledge when it shows up. According to Dr. Dan Siegel and Dr. Tina Payne Bryson, when we accurately tell ourselves we are experiencing an emotion ("I am feeling angry"), it helps to calm the "cortical firing" in our brains. They call the phenomenon "name it to tame it."

Study Your Angry Feelings

To effectively manage anger, we have to notice the physical sensations it creates in our bodies. This is similar to potty training. During potty training we learned to notice the sensations in our bladders or bowels and to link those sensations with words ("I have to pee or poop"), and then we learn to link those sensations with an action ("I therefore need to go to the bathroom"). What sensations do you notice arise in your body when anger is present? I notice that my temperature rises and I feel a bit sweaty. I also notice that my muscles and hands contract, and my jaw clenches.

Tolerate (Pause and Feel) Your Anger

This means instead of trying to eliminate our anger, we're trying to train ourselves to feel its presence in our bodies without reacting to it by either shutting it down or amplifying it. If we can allow ourselves to feel our anger without reacting to it, we can create the necessary pause that lets us *make decisions* instead of *having reactions.*

Excavate Your Anger

Researcher Brené Brown says that anger is a secondary emotion, meaning that where there's anger, other more vulnerable emotions and needs are also present. If we view anger as a helpful friend trying to point us toward or away from something, we can use it productively to support ourselves and our relationships rather than getting stuck and trying to blast our way through it. The simplest way to do this is to ask ourselves, *"What is this anger trying to help me see, or do, or release?"* I like to think of my anger as a lighthouse forewarning me about potential rocky shores that could wreck my boat, as well as guiding me toward the safe harbor of whatever it is I need.

Take Care of the Needs Beneath Your Anger

Once we have learned to notice our anger, tolerate the sensations that it brings to our bodies, and excavate our anger for needs, the next step in managing anger is to take action to meet the needs we excavated. In potty training this is the step when we walk our butts to the bathroom and put our waste where it belongs.

In the context of our underlying needs, that might be having a courageous conversation with someone about a change we need to see in our relationship with them. Or it might be going on a long run to stomp our anger through the pavement so we can get a release about things that we don't have the power to change. Or it might be gathering for a peaceful protest to share our anger with a collective voice.

Get Support

Sometimes our anger is so entrenched we need support to learn how to release it in healthy ways. Our anger might be a symptom of the fact that we are chronically depressed or anxious, or under the influence of unresolved trauma. This is a get-ourselves-into-therapy situation. Because anger that won't sit down is anger that needs a witness to help us figure out why it is so present in our lives.

Compassionate Self-Talk Scripts

- *"These feelings in my body mean that I'm angry, but they don't mean that I'm unsafe. I can tolerate the sensations while I listen to what they're telling me about what I need."*
- *"Underneath my anger is an unmet need to be discovered, and the more I listen to what I need, the less angry I will feel."*
- *"It is my responsibility to manage my anger no matter what triggered it."*

Trusty Tidbit

PASSING ON PASSIVE AGGRESSION

What we call passive aggression isn't actually passive. It's a covert attempt to communicate frustration and anger without taking ownership of the feelings. It's what we resort to when we haven't given ourselves full permission to be honest about our feelings and needs.

When I feel the urge to conceal my true feelings in passive packaging, I remind myself how confusing and jarring it feels to me when other people send obscure darts my way instead of being honest with me about why they are angry at me.

Sometimes we are angry at someone and don't know how to explain it to ourselves or to them, and if that's the case, we can use a placeholder statement like, "I'm having an angry response right now, and I am not sure why or what I need. Let me get clear on that and then I will let you know what I need from you."

Remember it's kind to be direct about our needs and feelings.

Further Reading

Anger: Wisdom for Cooling the Flames by Thich Nhat Hanh
Between Us: How Cultures Create Emotions by Batja Mesquita
The Dance of Anger by Harriet Lerner, PhD
The Relaxation and Stress Reduction Workbook by Martha Davis, PhD, Elizabeth Robbins Eshelman, MSW, and Matthew McKay, PhD

How to Deal with Feeling Anxious

"You don't have to control your thoughts; you just have to stop letting them control you."

—DAN MILLMAN, *Way of the Peaceful Warrior*

Feeling anxious is another feeling that all human beings contend with. And something that tends to increase once we have children.

Anxiety is a specialized form of fear. Pure fear is a body state we experience in the *presence* of danger or threat. For example if we encounter a snake in our backyard, fear is our nervous system's response to help us leap into action and escape from the snake. (Unless we're experienced snake handlers, and then I guess we'd feel excitement or endearment??? David Blaine, can you fact-check me here?)

Anxiety, on the other hand, is a state we experience when we *imagine* potential danger or a threat *in the future*. For example if we're inside our house and imagine there's a snake in our backyard, our bodies will still produce anxiety in response to the *thought of the snake*, even if no such snake exists.

Anxiety arises in our bodies as:

- Thoughts or images of unfortunate things happening
- Body sensations such as our hearts beating fast, finding it hard to catch our breath, or feeling shaky all over

Since the world is a place full of potential harm, our brains have evolved not only to react to present danger but also to anticipate potential future danger. Especially in response to our children's safety and well-being.

When our children are small we might experience anxiety as we imagine them falling into deep water or stepping onto a busy street. This anxiety can motivate us to get them into a life jacket or keep them close when cars are near. When they get to adolescence we might worry about them getting hurt in a car accident or being assaulted at a party. In these scenarios our anxiety can propel us to educate and equip our teens with the knowledge they need to stay safe.

In small doses *anxiety motivates us toward care and protection.*

When we experience anxiety of a low to moderate intensity and can manage our responses to it, it serves as a healthy source of energy to help us prepare for the future, execute tasks, and prevent discomfort or danger.

But, like anger, *unmanaged anxiety* can *cause* problems instead of preventing them.

How Unmanaged Anxiety Affects Our Children

When anxiety is chronically present or intrusively intense it doesn't improve anyone's safety; it decreases how safe we feel instead. And since our children look to us for safety cues, it can lead to them catching our anxiety or feeling responsible for calming us down. When anxiety has reached this level, it becomes *intrusive anxiety*.

- *"I feel anxious all the time."*
- *"I feel paralyzed by the intensity of anxiety I experience."*

Intrusive anxiety can put us in a frenzy of action, or it can paralyze us from action by flooding us with all the ways our next steps could end negatively.

Unlike a healthy dose of anxiety, intrusive anxiety distracts us from the things we can control, and it fixates our minds and thoughts on things we cannot.

Anxiety has become intrusive when:

- We are constantly anxious and focused on what could go wrong.
- We regularly share our anxious and intrusive thoughts with our children to try to help us feel better.
- We struggle to relax and are constantly moving, preparing, and planning because we start to panic if we sit still.
- We restrict our children's natural drive for greater independence out of fear.
- We point out risk factors so often that our children or teens don't feel safe anywhere in the world.
- We constantly check in with our children or teens about possible pain or suffering that they're feeling but not admitting.
- We hover over our children or teens in social settings instead of letting them learn, make their own decisions, and face their own mistakes.
- We are hypervigilant about not making a mistake (in any setting) and model extreme expectations of ourselves.
- We constantly correct our children.
- We obsess about time scarcity.
- We constantly over plan and run through our to-do lists.
- We're so fixated on our own anxiety that we don't take the time to listen to our children and hear how it is impacting them.

When we live in a constant state of intrusive anxiety, our children can't rely on us as a calming resource. Instead of feeling reassured when they're near us, they're infected by our anxious body states and mindsets (messing with gift #1, to feel we can handle what they feel).

This can create a repellent effect in some children. Instead of feeling drawn to us, their nervous systems push them away from us to avoid our anxiety. The more we try to pull them closer, the more they seek separation from us. Instead of feeling that we want them close (gift #3, they end up feeling that we want to control them or that we lack trust in their capacity).

Our anxious states can also have the opposite effect. Some of our children will catch our anxiety and will cling to our sides instead of exploring the world around them. They become enmeshed with us and lose the opportunity to fully develop their own sense of themselves and the world.

Whether our anxiety is propelling our children away from us or keeping them stuck by our sides, it's our job to work toward feeling more secure in ourselves and in the world around us so we can transfer that security to our children.

Anxiety is not a trait or a permanent condition; it's an emotional state, and with effort, can be reduced to levels that are helpful instead of harmful. This is *very* important to remember as we do this work because otherwise we can easily add a new worry—about our worrying habit—to our pile of anxiety.

Let's Grow!

We're all visited by anxious feelings from time to time, but here are a few ways to make sure the anxiety doesn't move in and overstay its welcome:

Personify a Wise Guide Character to Talk with Your Anxiety

Imagine a character that represents your inner wisdom. Have this character offer you warm understanding for what you are feeling. Then imagine them offering you reassurance about your capacity and your resources. Then ask your wise character to guide you to focus on the things you have control over and release the things you cannot influence.

Create an Anxiety Accountability Buddy

Find someone in your life who is wise and grounded and can be available to help you regulate your emotions and thoughts when you become anxious. Ask them to be someone in your life who helps you find your calm when you are stuck in an anxiety storm.

When my son was first born, Google News served me up a clickbait article about how to prevent playground kidnapping. The combination of persuasive writing and my sleep-deprived, hormone-doused brain allowed that article to push me into a pit of anxiety and preoccupation about all the ways a nefarious stranger could steal my child. I became obsessed with this scary thought and considered avoiding playgrounds altogether.

So I went to my husband and said, "I'm feeling very worried about playground kidnappings. Can you fact-check me here? What's a more likely scenario: our son getting kidnapped at a playground in the three seconds that I look away or our son losing trust in me as a reliable parent because I am constantly keeping him close and looking out for kidnappers?" He replied, "Number two, hands down." I'm so glad I let his reassurance take the reins. Because I am a parent who pays close attention, and living in fear of an unlikely kidnapping wasn't going to keep my child more safe, it was just going to keep us all more on edge.

Start Up a Meditation Habit

If you struggle to feel still or to rest in a safe moment, learning to meditate and use mindfulness practices can teach you to use information from the present moment to help you fight off unhelpful anxiety.

Reduce/Eliminate Caffeine Use

I know this piece of advice is a real killjoy. We love to love our coffee and tea. *But* we have solid evidence that caffeine can have a serious effect on our anxiety states. While it may not be fun to cut down on the java, it might be worth an experiment to see if it helps. Try dating decaf for a couple of weeks and report back.

Reduce/Eliminate Alcohol Use

Alcohol acts as a depressant in our nervous systems, and when depression visits, anxiety follows. Some of our bodies are more sensitive to mood changes from alcohol than others. Similar to the caffeine reduction, it could be worth slowing down your intake or taking some time off. (Note: If you drink a few drinks per day, consult with your health provider before going cold turkey off alcohol. There are some dangerous neurological side effects that can come with stopping too quickly without medical support.)

Consider Therapy, Medications, or Herbal Supports

Sometimes our anxiety is so ingrained that we need a little extra help to calm our nervous systems. If you've tried meditating, changing your caffeine and alcohol habits, talking with trusted people, and using guided visuals to help you reduce your anxiety, it could be time to seek out help from a professional, such as a therapist, doctor, herbalist, or acupuncturist.

Trusty Tidbit

GIVE YOUR ANXIETY A PET NAME

If you struggle with a regular presence of anxiety or panic, help your brain feel less worried about worrying by giving your anxiety a pet name.

My anxiety is named Janet. She really cares about me, but she's fairly dramatic and sometimes enters my brain without knocking first. I know Janet has taken over my brain when all the objects in my rearview mirror appear closer than they really are. In order to decrease her influence over me, I envision Janet biting her nails and rapidly sharing her catastrophic thoughts. Then I remember why I don't usually take advice from Janet. She's pretty intense. But I feel bad for her, so I imagine offering her a blanket and permission to binge-watch *The Fresh Prince of Bel-Air* until she feels calmer and more rational.

When we name our feeling states or find visuals to describe them (my friend's seven-year-old daughter calls her anxiety "the purple fuzzball"), it helps our brains to calm down and reset our perspective on the present moment.

Compassionate Self-Talk Scripts

- *"It's courageous to seek support and utilize resources to help me manage my anxiety. My ability to ask for help and to try support options is a sign of my resilience and strength."*
- *"This anxiety is loud in my head right now, but it's not my wise advisor and I don't have to believe what it's saying."*
- *"I'm capable of changing any habit I've formed over the years that has added to my anxious feelings and state of mind."*

- *"I deserve the time and investment that it takes to learn how to feel safe and calm and mindful of the moment I am in."*
- *"It is totally acceptable that I need support from other people when I'm feeling anxious and overwhelmed."*
- *"I can handle what's happening in my life right now. I'm capable of pausing and listening to my deepest wisdom and making the best next choice that I have available to me."*

Further Reading

Don't Believe Everything You Think by Joseph Nguyen
Raising Calm Kids in a World of Worry by Ashley Graber, LMFT, and Maria Evans, LMFT
Soothe Your Nerves: The Black Woman's Guide to Understanding and Overcoming Anxiety, Panic, and Fears by Angela Neal-Barnett
Stop Overthinking: 23 Techniques to Relieve Stress (video) by Nick Trenton
The Art of Letting Go by Nick Trenton
The Stress-Proof Brain by Melanie Greenberg, PhD

How to Deal with Feeling

At Odds with Our Children

"Never let a problem to be solved become more important than a person to be loved."
—BARBARA JOHNSON, *The Joy Journal*

Of all the various ways our parenting journeys can play out, there's one thing we'll all encounter as parents: the inevitable situation in which we find ourselves feeling at odds with our children. The question isn't whether we'll ever feel at odds with our children; it is what we'll feel at odds about. And to what degree?

These situations are usually small and benign initially, such as when our toddlers first dissent over bedtime, or when our elementary school children debate whether there should be a limit on the amount of time they spend watching *Bluey*. When we hit differences with our children at these ages, it's usually a struggle between their drive for autonomy and our role as their protector. But as our children grow into adolescents and young adults, our differences become more complex. And the reasons for those differences are no longer as simple as them pushing back their broccoli. Our children might start to challenge our biases, cultural practices, and deepest values and belief systems.

As a person who takes great joy in being my full, authentic self, it has been interesting to navigate the waters of tweenhood with my son. My desire to be silly and to sing and dance at all hours of the day creates serious discomfort in his nervous system. He feels exposed and panicky about my self-expression, giving me death stares when I make a mom joke or get groovy to some background music at the grocery store.

It can be truly discombobulating to us when our children feel differently than we do. Perhaps *they* love something that *we* don't (video games, anyone?). Or they're wired to feel emotions differently in their bodies (such as sensitivity levels). Or they may develop different views on the cosmos. These differences can put us into some real relational pickles.

Which is why it is our job to put in the work to respond as maturely as we can when the odds goombas start inching their way between us and our children.

How Chronically Being at Odds with Us Affects Our Children

How we handle our conflicts with our children will affect the way that our children feel when we are at odds with them. While conflict is inevitable in the parent-child relationship, the way we handle ourselves in that conflict can make a massive difference in how deeply it affects our children and our relationships with them.

The key is in responding from an emotionally regulated place and making connection and repairs as soon as we can.

When a disagreement with our children is chronic or prolonged, it compromises all five of the gifts of a secure parent. If we are constantly at odds, they cannot use our support, trust our delight, feel understood by us, or feel fully accepted by us.

Let's Grow!

The questions I ask myself when I'm feeling at odds with anyone in my brood are, "Who do I want to be in the face of these differences? And what memory do I want to make about my response to this situation?" While it stinks to be at odds with our children, it is par for the course, and if we approach the situation with our relationships in mind, the challenging moments can actually help us grow closer together. Here are some things to keep in mind as we face the odds:

Remembering What We Do and Do Not Have Control Over

We do not get to decide how our children feel, what they think, who or what they love, or what they will choose to do with their lives. This is so important to remember when we feel at odds with them because we can get distracted into trying to *control our children* and consequently lose control over *our relationships with them.*

If our goal is to have positive relationships with our children, then we want to be the kind of parents who can hold onto their hearts even when we are in a disagreement. We should address differences with openness, respect, humility, and collaborative problem-solving. We want to be parents who are both guides and learners.

When the Odds Are Ever in Their Favor, but They Don't See It That Way

When our children are at odds with us over things that could have serious negative effects on their health and safety, it's our job to maintain the necessary boundaries that they're disputing. "*Yes, you do have to go to sleep.*" "*Yes, you do have to brush your teeth.*" "*No you cannot snowboard off the roof*" "*No you cannot go to a party at a house where the parents are away for the night.*"

At first they will be mad and tell us that we are *the worst parents ever*. But if we keep our limits and boundaries based on their well-being, and we offer our children compassion for what they are feeling, our decision to be a thoughtful and engaged parent will cultivate trust. The vast majority of people do not grow up still upset that their parents made them wear a bike helmet, even if it caused a season of tantrums or felt incredibly uncool during their teenage years.

The key is to stay consistent with our decisions so that when our children oppose our limits or expectations, we don't wobble. The more confident and clear we are in our boundaries, the easier it is to offer compassion when our kids push up against them.

Holding a boundary and compassion at the same time sounds like:

"*It makes sense that you're disappointed that I won't let you jump off the roof. You were so excited about it. But it's my job to keep you safe, so I have to veto a potential broken bone under my watch.*"

When the Odds Are More Complicated

When the odds we feel with our children are not about health or safety, they get much messier.

The odds might be about:

- Our children relating differently to us than we related to our parents.
- Our children rejecting our cultural or faith values or traditions
- Our children forming close relationships with people we don't prefer or trust.
- Our children having different temperaments or needs than we do.
- Our children doing or saying things that are triggering our unresolved traumas.

No matter what underlying dynamic is cultivating the tension between us and our children, there are some principles we can follow to reduce the fallout and enhance the process of feeling reconnected and in sync.

Responding over Reacting

When we face a challenging feeling or behavior in our children, it is vital to remember first and foremost that it is our *children* we are facing. How we handle our children's feelings and perspectives in tricky moments will determine whether they come to us about their complicated needs in the future. If we react negatively as a pattern, they won't get gift #5 from us, to feel we accept all of who they are.

For this reason it is most effective to prioritize *empathetically responding* to our children's feelings during conflict and not *defensively reacting* to the emotions that the conflict creates inside of us. (If this is hard for you, check out the section on defensiveness on page 51 to get some tips on changing your body from defensive to receptive.)

No parent can do this all the time of course. Certain scenarios can really ruffle my feathers and get me to react from a rabid animal stance instead of responding from a reassuring parent stance. But, just like any skill we are trying to master, we can learn this skill and put in the repetitions it takes to master leading with *empathy* instead of *defense.*

This is especially important when our children are sharing with us things that they feel tender or upset about. If we jump in with opinions on what we think they should do, or how we think they should see something differently, we miss out on giving them gift #1, showing them that we can handle what they feel.

Our children don't share feelings with us to find out what we think; they share feelings with us to find out if we care about what they are feeling.

We want to ensure that we protect the position we hold as someone they share vulnerable truths with—even if those truths oppose how we usually think or operate.

It's not our job to tell our children what they feel is wrong. It's our job to work to understand what they're feeling and to be supportive as they figure out who they are and what matters to them.

Many aspects of our children's feelings toward us, themselves, and the world evolve as they develop. So how do we deal with the differences that don't evolve in the direction we hoped they would? The key is to learn to live with those differences and to ensure that our love and acceptance of our children outshines them.

Order of Operations for Effective Responding When at Odds:

1. Focus our energy on empathy and understanding (wait before giving advice).
2. Get curious about where *our* emotional reactions to the situation are coming from (focus on regulating our bodies and minds).

3. Seek wise counsel from people we trust to help us (get new perspectives).
4. Take any concerns or questions to our children to follow up on at a time when we can sense that they feel our love and can hear our feedback (guide, don't chide).

Accepting over Directing

At the end of the day, our children are different from us, so it makes perfect sense that they feel differently from us too. While we have some influence over them, especially when they're young, that doesn't mean that we get to decide who they are or how they operate. Instead we get to decide *who we are and how we choose to respond to them.* And if we're humble enough, our children can be incredible teachers in our lives, opening us up to new ideas and richer, broader ways of seeing and experiencing the world.

Learning to accept our children for who they are *right now* gives us a huge advantage in creating and keeping a positive relationship with them. When we focus on accepting our children and working to reduce any impulse to change them, we get to enjoy the type of relationship that all kids long to have with their parents—one in which their parents are truly in tune, understanding, and learning alongside them.

Dialoguing Instead of Monologuing

When we're at odds with our offspring, we can get caught up in an instinct to lecture. I really like to lecture my kids when I feel scared, tired, or angry. It's not fun to see our children working against the things we want for them or working toward things that we fear. It can be annoying, frustrating, and even painful.

When a dictator impulse arises inside us, we can forget that the most effective way to influence our children is to ensure that our interactions are truly two-directional.

I find this works best when I let my kids go first at moments of contention. Once I realize that my lecture is only making things worse, I pause and say, "I'm really not catching what you're trying to get me to understand, am I?" Instead of repeating what I want them to hear from me, I start repeating back to them what they're saying. As I get into a listening stance, they start to melt, and so do their words. We reach the tender spot of what they need me to get, and there's usually something quite profound for me to learn.

Once we've melted into a connected state, I ask, "Do you feel heard by me now?" and look for an emphatic "yes" before I proceed to share some of my thoughts. And when I do share my thoughts, I make sure to keep us in dialogue mode by saying things like, "I am curious what you have to say about this idea," or "I may not be able to shift in the exact way you want me to, but I wonder if we can brainstorm other ways to make this feel less painful or uncomfortable?"

If we want to be securely connected to our children we need to spend as much time listening as we do sharing our thoughts and feelings.

Move Toward Presence, Not Panic

It can feel scary when we're at odds with our children. It's easy to become worried about their futures or our future relationships with them.

Unfortunately a panicked response to being at odds with them actually exacerbates the disconnection. The further we flail into our anxiety the less of a comforting presence we have to offer our children.

Instead of focusing on thoughts and feelings about how this moment could spiral into a dark and dreary future, we need to put Janet (the name I gave my anxiety) into a time-out and remember that our children need our confidence in the connection more than they need us to have a conflict-free relationship.

Getting out of sync with our children is normal. Having different opinions, values, and patterns is part of the process. When we choose to trust ourselves and our kids, those moments become opportunities for learning instead of liabilities. When we show up and say, "I'm here for you even though we are currently at odds," we can move from disagreement to deep connection, even if things turn out differently from how we'd imagined them.

Trusty Tidbit
COMMENTING ON THE CONFLICT

One of my favorite things to say to my kids during a fight is:

"I hate fighting with you because I love being connected to you. I don't know exactly how we're going to get ourselves out of this pickle, but I know for sure that we will."

Letting my kids know that I do not enjoy our disconnection helps them to trust that I'm working to reconnect with them and not simply trying to push my own agenda. (Sometimes it takes a good night's sleep to fully convince them of course.)

Compassionate Self-Talk Scripts

- *"It's challenging to feel at odds with my child, but that doesn't mean that my child is a challenge."*
- *"I don't know how to handle this situation yet, but I can use my heart to listen to my child, which will help me get clarity on what choices are right for both of us."*
- *"If I know that my expectations are going to help keep my child safe, healthy, and connected, it's okay if they don't currently understand or agree with me; in the long run, they will grow to trust that this was the right choice."*
- *"It's okay if my child is right, and I'm learning something new. Parenting is a developmental process too."*
- *"The bond I share with my child is more powerful than any struggle we have to navigate on this journey."*

Further Reading

All About Love by bell hooks

How to Talk So Kids Will Listen & Listen So Kids Will Talk by Adele Faber and Elaine Mazlish

Raising Children Compassionately by Marshall B. Rosenberg, PhD

Raising Kids with Big, Baffling Behaviors by Robyn Gobbel

Raising Securely Attached Kids by Eli Harwood

The Power of Showing Up: How Parental Presence Shapes Who Our Kids Become and How Their Brains Get Tired by Daniel Siegel, MD and Tina Payne Bryson PhD

How to Deal with Feeling

Body Disgust

"Our unapologetic embrace of our bodies gives others permission to unapologetically embrace theirs."
—SONYA RENEE TAYLOR, *The Body Is Not an Apology*

I'm pretty convinced that there are a total of about three people on earth who make it through their lives without having to contend with some form of body insecurity, disgust, or contempt. I can't prove that these people are real because they must have grown up on an obscure island isolated from emotional pain, exposure to marketing, generational trauma, and all forms of social oppression. But I guess they could exist. Either way, they aren't you or me.

Body disgust sounds like *my body (or someone else's body) is:*

- Too big
- Too small
- Too dark
- Too pale
- Too lumpy
- Too fat
- Too weak
- Too tall
- Too short
- Too curvy
- Too flat
- Too soft

- Too bulky
- Too sensitive
- Inadequate
- Undeserving of rest
- Undeserving of nourishment
- Undeserving of love, affection, and acceptance
- The wrong shape or has the wrong features
- Broken
- Wrong for something it feels
- Wrong for something it does
- Unworthy because it doesn't have a particular part or feature
- Unworthy because it isn't capable of a particular action or function

We can feel disgust toward our bodies for how they look, feel, or function. It's important to note that disgust at our bodies is *learned* and not innate. We learn to value (or devalue) our bodies as a result of our relationships with family members, peers, the cultures we live in, and the media we consume.

We may not be able to prevent our children from learning body disgust from outside sources, but we can certainly work on being a space where they learn to love their bodies as a way to help them fight the pressure to hate them.

Examples of Body Disgust in Parenting

- Looking at ourselves in mirrors or pictures and grimacing or insulting our bodies ("Ewwww, I look disgusting!")
- Constantly hiding our bodies or refusing to go swimming or enjoy outdoor activities, joking or berating ourselves that "no one needs to see this"
- Dieting regularly as an attempt to lose or gain weight to the level that we are more focused on changing our bodies than enjoying time with our children and other important people

- Making negative comments about other people's bodies, either in real life or portrayed in film, print, or online
- Idealizing certain body types and praising people who look a certain way or are a certain size
- Cultivating food fears via extreme dieting
- Being preoccupied with trying to change the way we appear, even when it causes us financial strain or time drain
- Comparing bodies and using appearances or physical performance to assess someone's primary value
- Denying our bodies the release, rest, or nourishment they need and encouraging our children or teens to do the same

How Our Feelings of Body Disgust Affect Our Children

It all depends on how chronic and loud our disgust toward our bodies is. Being stuck in feelings of consistent hatred about our bodies and vocalizing the disgust we feel toward ourselves ("Watch out, your fat cow of a mom is coming by" or "One of these days I will get my lazy butt to do something for once") harms our children in two significant ways:

1. It teaches them that bodies are only valuable when they fit specific criteria, which makes it more likely they'll find something to feel disgusted about concerning their own bodies.
2. It teaches them how to treat their bodies and other comparable bodies, potentially leading them to look down on people whose bodies are similar to theirs.

The judgments we make about our bodies become mental templates for our children and affect whether they learn to love or detest the skin they are in.

If we can find ways to express gratitude for our bodies (as imperfect as they may feel to us) and to take care of them, we can give our children a fighting chance to carry less generational body hatred than we have carried.

Body Disgust Doesn't Promote Health

Hating our bodies doesn't help us to become healthier, happier, more valuable, or more connected to others. (Though many marketing campaigns would love to differ with me on this to sell their products.)

When I was young I thought I would feel less self-disgust if my body looked a particular way. I even named my cat "Crystal Light" because I was so enamored by the confidence that the women in their magazine ads beamed from the pages. They were happy! Because they were thin! They were thin because they drank diet lemonade! The diet culture messaging came through so loud and clear for me that I wanted the product they were selling not only for myself but also for my cat.

But age and a solid amount of therapy (on both sides of the couch) have taught me that *the more we tell ourselves our bodies are wrong, the worse we feel about ourselves and the less likely we are to take action toward actual self-care.*

We can't hate our bodies into being something we love.

Instead we have to change what we believe it is about our bodies that makes them valuable.

Our bodies are valuable because they give us life. They give us connection and the opportunity to be a part of this precious human experiment that we're all in together.

STOP

Body disgust can trigger disordered eating, which can result in serious health concerns. If you're restricting calories, bingeing or purging food, exercising excessively, or feeling generally uncomfortable about your behavior in relation to food or exercise, please contact a health care professional who can find you the right help.

The opposite of body hatred isn't believing that we're beautiful or that our bodies are flawless; it's *believing that our presence is more valuable than our appearance.* And when we believe that our presence is what makes us valuable, it makes it far easier to love and care for ourselves.

Healthy habits develop from a healthy appreciation for our intrinsic value, not pressure to fit into a teeny tiny bikini or idealized standards of beauty.

When we value our bodies for their presence ("I am here!") and take practical actions to care for them, it helps us release old habits of scrutiny, shame, and harshness. When we view our bodies as gifts of life and not problems to be solved, we can live more fully and love more freely.

Body Disgust Has History

Trauma can produce feelings of body disgust. That trauma can come from two different, but detrimental sources.

Some of the trauma roots are personal, coming from our own lived experiences of physical, emotional, or sexual abuse. Harmful treatment by other people affects how we feel about our bodies.

A heartbreaking and common side effect of experiencing abuse is believing that we deserved what happened to us, or that our body became shamefully damaged as a result of the trauma we endured. But no*body* deserves to be mistreated, and every*body* deserves healing and respect no matter what we have gone through.

The problem is never our bodies; it is the *beliefs that people who abused us held about our bodies* and used to justify their mistreatment of us.

Body disgust can also grow from the roots of generational and cultural traumas. These disgust roots were initially planted in historical dynamics that have shaped our shared human history and stem from various misguided (at best) or dehumanizing (at worst) beliefs, including:

- That women's bodies are less valuable than men's bodies
- That bodies with dark skin are less valuable than bodies with light skin
- That heterosexual bodies are working properly, but LGBTQ bodies are broken or wrong for what they feel
- That someone who is particularly able is more valuable than someone who is differently abled
- That a body that has legal status has more value than a body that does not have legal status

Even though we've all been exposed to these historical beliefs, we don't have to allow them authority over the way we view our bodies or other people's. We can recognize that any message telling us that one body is more valuable than another is inherited from traumatic horsesh*t. We can replace those antiquated ideas with a passionate dedication to the belief that everyone's bodies are magical and valuable.

STOPPING THE TRADITION OF INHERITED BODY DISGUST

When we feel disgust toward our bodies, we're disconnecting from how our bodies actually feel and connecting to how other people think our bodies should feel or should make them feel.

Growing up, I heard my elders say things like "A moment on the lips, a lifetime on the hips" and "Nothing tastes as good as skinny feels." I watched smart, beautiful women struggling with extreme diets and beating themselves up for not meeting a particular vision of beauty. They didn't do this because it made them feel good; they did it because they were taught that feeling good mattered far less than looking good.

Unfortunately these family messages seeped into my own consciousness and joined the Crystal Light ads in my understanding of my own body. What was happening in my family aligned with the problematic messages I received from the wider world.

I know that my children, especially my daughters, will be exposed to these messages and will at some point experience these feelings. I hope that body disgust and diet culture will feel jarring and problematic to them rather than familiar. I believe that body disgust should not take up even a fraction of the space and energy it took up in my life or the lives of previous generations. We can do this. We can change the way we talk about our bodies, treat our bodies, and conceptualize the value of our bodies.

Let's Grow!

If you inhabit a body that has been labeled "lesser" as a result of cultural and historical trauma, I encourage you to embrace your anger and grief about this deception. It's unfair and cruel that you were taught to hate your body because of your gender, racial or ethnic identity, or sexual preferences. (I found some release in feeling angry and sad about the ways that messages toward my female body have made me want to shrink my size instead of taking up space.)

If your body has elements that are viewed as particularly valuable (and you view different bodies as lesser), you should consider how those beliefs have robbed you of a greater connection with the people in your life and wider community. (If the majority of films we watch, stories we read, and leaders we see in charge are people who experience the world like us, we miss out on huge swaths of the human experience by not hearing from those who don't have the same advantages.)

When body disgust arises, the ideal response is to offer ourselves compassion—body disgust is a horrible feeling. Our next job is to align with our bodies. To care for them, speak well of them, and listen closely to all the wisdom they have to share with us about how to live well in the world. Here are some helpful practices to help us all deepen our love for our bodies:

The Daily Love Note

Get a pad of sticky notes and make it a practice to write down something nice about your body every morning. Put the notes up on your bathroom mirror so you can absorb the love several times a day.

Trusty Tidbit
PROMOTING PEACE

Glennon Doyle blew my mind when she said, "There are two different ways to view the phrase 'making peace with our bodies.' The first is the labor we do to accept and love our bodies as they are. The second is the ways that we use our bodies to help promote peace in the world around us."

I've found that when we're stuck battling self-disgust, sometimes the most effective antidote is to focus our attention away from evaluating our bodies and onto the efforts we can make to care for other people's bodies instead. Activities such as volunteering, caregiving, protesting, advocating, and donating our money and time to causes we feel in our hearts. By advocating for peace in the world outside our body image battles, we can more easily detangle ourselves from the webs of self-contempt.

Follow the Thumper Rule

In the movie *Bambi*, the young deer's rabbit friend says, "If you can't say something nice, don't say nothing at all." Learning to love our bodies can be a complex process, but committing to not giving the mean words airtime can be simple. Make it a rule to no longer say unkind words about your body or anyone else's. If you're struggling with feeling awful for some reason, instead of saying, "*My body is gross*," say, "I'm feeling disconnected from my body's magic. I know it is still there; I'm just struggling to feel it."

Then take a minute to say some kind things to yourself about your body. For example:

- *"My eyes are such incredible helpers when I need to see things."*
- *"My ears let me listen to the music that soothes my soul."*
- *"My arms are so good at hugging."*

When we pause and pay attention to what our bodies are offering us, it can help us learn to love them more. We should focus on the things our bodies do to help us and not on how they look or perform for others.

Nourish

It's important to intentionally feed our bodies foods that give us energy, nutrients, and joy. When we offer our bodies nourishment, we're giving them what they need to run optimally. Sometimes that means prioritizing nutritious fruits and vegetables, and sometimes it means choosing more fun foods such as donuts and mochi. Either way, when you're nourishing your body, pay attention to what you're feeling and let yourself enjoy the experience.

Nurture

When we nurture our bodies, it helps our brains regulate, which helps to reduce our stress hormones and keeps us feeling better, both physically and emotionally. Nurture can involve small gestures, such as offering ourselves a moment of pleasure, like smelling something we love, or larger actions, such as taking a couple of days' holiday to rest and revive ourselves after a stressful period. Nurture looks different for everyone, but it works in the same way. The more we nurture ourselves, the more worthy we feel, and the more worthy we feel, the more likely we are to continue nurturing ourselves.

Trusty Tidbit
OUR BODIES ARE WONDERLANDS

One of my favorite things to do in rebellion against body disgust is to wonder out loud about my body in front of my kids (I wonder about theirs too).

- "I can't believe that there's a tiny little machine inside my ear that captures vibrations and translates them to my brain so that I can experience the sounds of your incredible laughter."
- "Isn't it incredible that this tiny little pinky toe plays a massive role in keeping me balanced? Without this wee little stub, I'd be wobbling around with sea legs."
- "You know what's crazy? I never have to tell my heart what to do; it just knows. Pumping blood through my body all day long. That's wild!"

When we wonder at our bodies, not just how they appear but the ways they keep us alive, it helps our children see more about their bodies than how attractive they are for others to look at.

Change Our Image Inputs

The images we consume can impact how we feel about our bodies. If we're on social media, scrolling through doctored images of people who work out for a living, we're likely to experience a higher dose of body disgust. Next time you're on social media, check the accounts you follow that trigger increased body disgust for you and either unfollow or mute them. Then intentionally follow people who promote body positivity and who inspire you to be kinder toward yourself.

Compassionate Self-Talk Scripts

- *"My body is incredible and it deserves to be heard and appreciated."*
- *"Every part of my body deserves to be loved and spoken to with kindness."*
- *"My body works hard to take care of me twenty-four seven, and I can return that favor by nurturing myself in ways that feel kind and caring to me."*
- *"One of the kindest things I can do for my body is to offer myself things that help me feel good and nourished."*
- *"I'm feeling some painful shame about my body right now, but feelings like this are never facts."*

Further Reading

Body Happy Kids: How to Help Children and Teens Love the Skin They're In by Molly Forbes

Body Neutral: A Revolutionary Guide to Overcoming Body Image Issues by Jessi Kneeland

Daring Greatly by Brené Brown

Decolonizing the Body: Healing, Body-Centered Practices for Women of Color to Reclaim Confidence, Dignity, and Self-Worth by Kelsey Blackwell

Fat Chance, Charlie Vega by Crystal Maldonado

More Than A Body: Your Body Is an Instrument, Not an Ornament by Lexie Kite and Lindsay Kite

The Body Is Not an Apology: The Power of Radical Self-Love by Sonya Renee Taylor

The Eating Instinct: Food Culture, Body Image, and Guilt in America by Virginia Sole-Smith

You Have the Right to Remain Fat by Virgie Tomar

How to Deal with Feeling Defensive

"Openness may not completely disarm prejudice,
but it's a good place to start."

—**JASON COLLINS**, *Why NBA Center Jason Collins Is Coming Out Now*

We all have an inbuilt instinct to defend ourselves in order to survive potential threats and attacks. Our defensive feelings are valuable and necessary when we're truly at risk: defensiveness can be positive when it actually serves to *protect us.*

I can think of many times that defensiveness has arisen in my body to help me and the people I love. The time in junior high school when a group of boys started harassing me and tried to grab me inappropriately while I was trick-or-treating in a friend's neighborhood. The defensive feelings that arose in my body helped me stand up for myself and use my pillowcase of candy as a shield and a weapon until they eventually left me alone. Defensiveness served me well that day.

Or when my husband and his best friend were on a ferry in Indonesia, and a group of men with automatic weapons on the boat stared at them menacingly and then followed them around for the entire overnight voyage. They naturally felt on guard and defensive, and this motivated them to strategically move as close to the exit as possible for docking. When the boat reached its destination, the men attempted to kidnap them. They defended themselves and bolted into a taxi, where they immediately locked the doors, narrowly escaping as the brave taxi driver put his pedal to the metal and screeched out of the loading zone. Defensiveness at its finest.

Had they not felt defensive and had the instinct to fight for their escape, I wonder if I would be holding my sweetheart today. (Also—important note—my husband thinks I wrote this story as too much of a "thriller" when it was more of a "suspense" experience!)

If something or someone is truly getting in the way of our safety, then the defensive signals in our bodies can help protect us. But this instinct toward defensiveness can be problematic when it becomes a habit or when it arises in situations where we're safe and are being offered opportunities for support and growth.

Situations Where Defensive Feelings Create Problems Instead of Solving Them

- When we argue against feedback instead of trying to hear what someone needs
- When we're on the lookout for ways that people misunderstand us
- When we get physically tense or triggered in discussions about ideas or plans
- When we believe that anyone who thinks differently from us is attacking us by doing so
- When we're unwilling to listen to or attempt to understand other people's ways of thinking, believing, or doing
- When we struggle to feel safe in deep conversations with people who love us

How Our Chronic Defensive Responses Can Affect Our Children

When we have a defensiveness problem, it's hard for our children to give us authentic feedback about what they need from us (getting in the way of gift #1, feeling that we can handle what they feel). This makes it hard for them to continue seeking closeness to us over time because things between us become unresolved (getting in the way of gift #3, sensing that we want to have a close relationship with them).

Even if we're generally loving and caring, if we can't handle feedback without getting prickly or arguing against it, our children will develop defensiveness in response to our defensiveness, making it nearly impossible for them to feel fully securely connected to us (getting in the way of gift #2, feeling that we understand them).

Some of our children will inherit our defensive habits and spar with us directly when we attempt to give them feedback. Others will forgo their needs and side with us, choosing a people-pleasing approach (see page 224) to cope with our defensiveness, leaving them disconnected from their own needs in an attempt to stay connected to us (getting in the way of gift #5, feeling that we fully accept them for who they are, which includes how they feel in their relationship with us).

Examples of Problematic Defensiveness in Parenting

We all get defensive from time to time with our children. The problem arises when defensiveness is chronic and unresolved.

Problematic defensiveness toward our children looks like:

- Jumping to justify our actions instead of being curious and open to hearing our children's explanations about how they made them feel
- Denying something that we did or didn't do instead of taking ownership
- *Blaming our children* for having needs instead of hearing what they are trying to tell us
- Blaming someone else defensively to reverse the attention when we're called out

Let's Grow!

When we notice that defensive feelings are becoming a problem for us or our children, our growth path is to learn how to dial down defensiveness by increasing receptiveness.

Receptivity is a fancy word to describe the ability to *receive* someone else's emotions, perspectives, or needs without shutting down or blowing up. On a physical level, receptivity is about letting our guard down and opening up our hearts to fully hear what is being shared with us so that we can care more deeply for that person and strengthen our connection with them.

In secure parenting, this is a *must learn* and *continually practice* type skill.

Receptivity is central to creating secure relationships, and without it, we can almost guarantee that as our children grow, so will their instinct to grow emotionally distant from us.

Find a Receptivity Mentor

This could be someone you know in real life or a character in a book or film. Look for someone who remains calm and open when receiving feedback. Someone who has a warm demeanor and is relationally oriented. Study their mindsets. What is it they prioritize? What do they believe about themselves? What are their beliefs about their duties to others? How do they treat their bodies and their time? Let them teach you the way of receptivity.

Make a Defense Op Plan

Get a sheet of paper and write down all the scenarios that you think deserve a defensive response from you. For example, if someone is trying to steal your car. My husband once caught someone trying to steal his car, and he confronted them and chased them down the street successfully. That's a great example of an appropriate defensive response! List as many situations as you need to.

Then on another piece of paper, write out all the scenarios in which you want to be receptive. And especially important, the relationships where you want close secure bonds. These are the people who deserve all of your efforts to be intentionally receptive.

Keep these two papers somewhere in your home where you can regularly see them and remind yourself about who, when, why, and what deserves your defense response, and who, when, why, and what deserves your efforts to keep your defenses low and your heart open.

Master the Pause

If getting defensive is a long-term habit for us, the gap between that habit and learning to be open and receptive can feel like a very large chasm. But it isn't as large a gap as it may seem, and the best way to shrink it is to learn how to pause when we notice defensive feelings arising inside of us. Work to practice pausing throughout your day in conversations or actions and saying out loud or in your head, "I need a minute to figure out what I want my next response to be."

Pausing gives our brains the extra time they need to register safety and to send in calming neurotransmitters to help us access our thinking brains. The pause is often the only solution we need because once we've paused instead of reacting, it becomes *far* easier to respond with receptivity instead of defense.

Open Up Them Heart Gates

Intentionally sharing our hearts with people who are genuinely caring helps us to feel safer in the world, which helps us to be less defensive. If this is hard for you, you've likely had some relationship trauma in your life that has led you to keep your emotional cards close to your chest. That makes sense. Keep your eyes peeled though for people who are capable of handling your cards with care. They are out there—keep looking and you will find them.

Compassionate Self-Talk Scripts

- *"I deserve to be loved and fully known, just like every other human being."*
- *"It feels scary to live without my guard up, but I am capable of becoming someone who is far more open and connected."*
- *"I don't have to react immediately to everything, especially when I'm feeling triggered, overwhelmed, or anxious. I can give myself a moment to pause and find my bearings instead of reacting before I've had time to assess."*

- *"It's normal that I feel defensive in situations where I'm truly being threatened, but I can learn to let go in places where I am safe and loved."*

> ***Trusty Tidbit***
>
> **TIME-OUT**
>
> When I'm feeling defensive and I can tell that my energy is ping-ponging back and forth with one of my children, I find it incredibly helpful to put myself in a time-out. I say something like, "I need someone to put me in a time-out until I can find my calm brain and use my gentle words!!!"
>
> By poking fun at my defensiveness, even just a little bit, it helps me release it more fully and return to the more receptive and regulated state that I need to think clearly and connect effectively.
>
> My kids also really love the opportunity to banish me for a bit. Rude but understandable.

Further Reading

How to Listen, Hear, and Validate: Break Through Invisible Barriers and Transform Your Relationships by Patrick King

I Never Thought of It That Way: How to Have Fearlessly Curious Conversations in Dangerously Divided Times by Monica Guzmán

Triggers: How We Can Stop Reacting and Start Healing by David Richo

You're Not Listening: What You're Missing and Why It Matters by Kate Murphy

How to Deal with Feeling

Jealous of Our Children

"Learning not to envy someone else's blessing is what grace looks like."

—RUPI KAUR, *The Sun and Her Flowers*

Although feeling jealous or envious of our children is not something we usually admit to others. Just as we can feel anger or sadness in response to our children, we can also be visited by feelings of envy and jealousy.

We might feel envious of the privileges our children experience that we didn't have as we grew up. Or jealous of the close relationships they've built that give them a sense of belonging that we never had. Or envious of the youth, beauty, talent, or confidence they possess that we do not.

Envy and jealousy are painful feelings in any situation, but they're worse when they're connected to our children. Because if we're aware we're feeling those emotions, we're usually also visited by a heaped helping of shame. ("What's wrong with me that I'm feeling this way? How could I do this to my child???")

And if we don't know how to handle the shame, it can get curdled into contempt and projected onto our children. "*What's wrong with them? It's their fault I'm feeling this way!!*"

If you've ever gone through that painful pipeline from jealousy to shame to contempt, you're not alone. And I'd like to clarify something: *feeling jealous of our children* is very different from *acting out our jealous feelings toward them.*

Every parent goes through these feelings at some level. The level at which we struggle with jealousy toward our children is related to what we lacked in our childhood, especially in the most important realms: attention, soothing, adoration, delight, belonging, safety, practical support, and emotional care.

I had a moment when I was buying my son a pair of brand-name shoes that he wanted. He was *so* giddy and appreciative that even though I was excited for him, I noticed a pang of jealousy arise in my body. I couldn't remember a moment quite like it in my own childhood. I could remember that my mom was an exclusive discount footwear shopper, and that if I wanted shoes with a brand name (a.k.a. cool), I had to babysit my way to buying them. (And given the babysitting rates I charged in the '90s, this meant more work than I could usually get my hands on.)

As a kid (and still to this day), fashion was a significant form of my self-expression. While I appreciate my mother's frugal approach to footwear now, the younger me longed for a world where my mom recognized that branded shoes were a big deal in my social circle.

This moment of jealousy had no impact at all on my son, and unless he reads this book as an adult, he'll never even know it happened. But it certainly had me wondering if there was something deeper at play for me besides shoe shopping.

How Our Jealousy of Our Children Affects Them

It is fundamentally confusing for a child to feel and process jealous feelings from a parent. This is an area that can damage all five gifts we're trying to offer to our children (page x). If they come face-to-face with our jealous feelings, it makes it feel unsafe to share their celebrations with us (gift #4). It also affects their sense of being understood by us (gift #2) because they had no intention of triggering jealous feelings inside of us.

It also collapses their ability to sense our desire to be close to them (gift #3) because they can tell that we're experiencing negative emotions as a result of their positive attributes or circumstances. And this gets in the way of them perceiving that we find them delightful. Instead they sense that we're threatened by the good things in their lives. This also gets in the way of them feeling we can show up for them (gift #4) and that we fully accept them (gift #5) because our negative, envious state shows otherwise.

Let's Grow!

The emotionally mature response to feeling jealous or envious of our children is to manage our feelings by resisting the urge to project them and learning to reflect on them instead. In my shoe scenario, the projection would have been me saying something like, "Must be nice to have a mom who will buy you the shoes you want; my mom would never have paid for me to get shoes this fancy." Or worse, teasing him for his need to have "cool shoes" and taking down his joy with a spark of mockery.

Reflection Protection

The healthy way to get relief from jealousy and envy is through self-reflection. Instead of asking our children to hold our messy responses to them, we can shift the attention toward ourselves and dive deeper into what we're processing. For me, that deeper dive was reflecting on what my childhood was like beyond the actual shoe situation. It was acknowledging that my parents were treading water in many ways, sometimes financially and usually emotionally. As I reflected on what I was feeling in that tween stage of my adolescence, I realized that my childhood often felt serious and worrisome. There hadn't been a ton of room for the fluffy stuff of life, including cool shoes.

My jealousy in that moment had more to do with my younger self longing for my parents to be stable enough for a little indulgence. A little more "for the fun of it" and a little less "what if we run out of money or get divorced?"

Grief almost always lies beneath jealousy and envy. For me the grief entirely relieved the envy, and laid a beautiful opening for me to feel thankful that I could give my son a facet of childhood I hadn't experienced at the same intensity.

What if that reflection process had not relieved my feelings of envy toward my son? Then I would have marched my butt into conversations with my sweetheart, my therapist, and my close friends so the caring adults in my life could help me process the grief underlying the jealous feelings. Jealousy and envy are lighthouses for unprocessed grief from the past or unmet needs in the present.

Trusty Tidbit
PARENT YOUR INNER CHILD

When you notice that you're feeling jealous toward your children, envision giving what they have to your younger self who wanted or needed it.

Let's say you're jealous because your children are close to their father, and that's something you never had. Close your eyes and picture yourself at the age at which you feel you most needed a close relationship with your father. Then imagine the father you wished could have been there. It could be a mature version of your real-life father, someone you know, or even a fictional character. (For me it's Michael Landon playing Charles Ingalls in *Little House on the Prairie*.)

Let that vision play until you cry and feel a bit better. Give yourself the feeling that you longed to have from the thing you never got. It will make it much easier to celebrate the fantastic reality that your children actually have what you didn't.

Rejecting a Legacy of Jealousy

I asked my friend Diana to share how her mother's unexamined jealousy of her had affected her, and how she stopped the cycle with her own children.

> When I was growing up, "They're just jealous" was my mom's favorite refrain for any conflict I had with a friend. It never quite fit most of the situations I was dealing with. It did, however, fit another situation well: my relationship with her. She frequently didn't seem to take pride in my accomplishments. She rarely praised me for my achievements, or worse, compared them to

her own. She too often took little interest in my awards or special events as a child.

The impact on my life and my relationships was lasting and painful. For a long time, I struggled with being a chronic overachiever. I sought out unhealthy forms of validation and constantly questioned my own self-worth, always wondering if I was enough. In my relationship with her, I remain guarded in sharing much of anything, knowing that even now, I can't always trust her to see me with an open heart and mind. Though I have sought healing through therapy and feel like I am a mostly happy and healthy adult, the hurt still lingers.

I now realize the pain behind my mother's jealousy. I see how, as a single mother who experienced traumatic things herself growing up, she fought to provide me with more opportunities than she ever had. As a child, I was incapable of—and not responsible for—being grateful to her. But it must have been hard for her to sacrifice so much and be largely unappreciated. And I suspect she was afraid that the success she was working so hard to make possible for me would ultimately distance me from her.

When my own daughter was small, I started to notice similar feelings. I got curious. Was there some part of me that wished I had my daughter's freedom? Her creativity? Her joy? In those moments, I learned to find ways to offer myself more of those things while celebrating that she was thriving. Wasn't that what I wanted? I discovered that it was. I learned that beneath the jealousy, what I was really feeling was grief. Grief for myself as a child. And fear that if I wasn't hard on her, the world would be harder. Those feelings may have been what drove my mother too. But they didn't (and don't) serve me or my relationship to my daughter. It was that reminder that gave me the compassion and the courage to choose differently.

A NOTE ON NARCISSISM

If you struggle from time to time with feeling jealous of your children or their lives, it doesn't automatically mean you are a narcissist. If you grew up with a narcissistic parent it is normal to worry that you could have that struggle too. Why? Because it was deeply traumatic to be in the care of someone who couldn't hold onto your mind and heart at the same time they held onto theirs.

It makes sense that you do not want to pass on this reality to your children, and that your worry about this keeps you up at night. ("Did I act just like my mother?" "Was I doing the same thing to my child that my dad did to me?" "How do I know???")

The fact that you're worried about it is a very promising sign that you're not suffering from the same mindsets that your parents did. When someone is in a narcissistic pattern, they're unable to tolerate the idea that they could be wrong or fallible. That means they did not lie awake at night worrying about whether or not they were narcissistic toward you.

Narcissism is the presence of obsessive selfishness and the absence of dedicated care for others. The presence of *some* selfishness or periodic failures of empathy does not equal narcissism. It equals humanity. Get good at apologizing (see Trusty Tidbit Tips for Effective Apologies on page 16), and continue to learn.

Remember that if we struggle with immaturity from time to time, but *we take accountability for that and work to improve*, we're not acting narcissistically. We're just on a growth journey.

The more willing we are to acknowledge our areas of growth without collapsing in shame or deflecting with blame, the less narcissistic we are.

You're Not JUST Jealous

The most important thing to do when we feel jealous of our children is to dig deeper to figure out what's triggering the envy. The feelings are not actually about our children and are not *just* anything. They are meaningful signals illuminating a healing path for us. Our jealous feelings reveal issues from our past that need our acknowledgment and compassion.

Compassionate Self-Talk Scripts

- *"It's okay that I'm feeling jealous of my children. That doesn't make me a bad parent or even put my kids in a weird position. My job is to make sure I don't project the mess onto them and instead work through these feelings with the adults in my life who are committed to supporting me."*
- *"I can feel envious and still feel grateful that my children have wonderful qualities or advantages in their lives."*
- *"These feelings are not facts about my character; they're lighthouses letting me know where I have unresolved grief."*
- *"This jealous feeling is inviting me to understand something about my past or my present and to let out the grief and pain related to it."*

Further Reading

I'm Happy for You (Sort Of . . . Not Really): Finding Contentment in a Culture of Comparison by Kay Wills Wyma

Radical Acceptance by Tara Brach

The Art of Letting Go by Nick Trenton

Why Has Nobody Told Me This Before? by Dr. Julie Smith

How to Deal with Feeling **Judged**

"Do you see me? This is the big question your child is asking every day. Can you recognize me for who I am, different from your dreams and expectations for me, separate from your agenda for me?"

—DR. SHEFALI TSABARY, *The Awakened Family*

It can be challenging at times to accurately see and understand our children, even when we're alone with them. But to make it even trickier for everyone involved, we also have to navigate the inevitability of other people judging our children or our responses to them. Judgment might come from a stranger on an airplane, a close friend, or a family member. Or, to keep things exciting, it might come from inside our imaginations!

Whether we're encountering actual judgment from others or imagined judgment in our minds, how we respond to these feelings can have a far-reaching impact on us and our kids.

How Does Being Preoccupied with Other People's Judgments Affect Our Children?

Since we have limited amounts of attention and energy, focusing on other people's judgments directly affects the amount of time and energy we have to give our children what they need from us (taking away from gift #3, our children feeling that we want to be close to them). Of course we all feel judged at times, and that's not in and of itself a problem for our children. They feel judged at times too. The problem is when we become preoccupied with a real or perceived judgment.

We can also count on other people's judgments to be a distraction from goal #5, for our children to feel that we accept them for their full, authentic selves. When we're absorbed in what other people think about our children or our parenting, our kids can sense our anxiety and feel pressure to hide their truest selves to protect them or protect us.

This preoccupied state can also get in the way of our children feeling pride and delight from us, which compromises gift #4, our kids knowing that we will show up for them. Instead of being present for their little victories, we become entangled in fear over what other people think they should be doing or becoming.

If we fixate on the opinions of onlookers, we're likely out of sync with our children's experiences, and that makes it hard for us to cheer them on in the way they need.

Our goal is to learn how to manage the discomfort and distraction that comes with feeling judged.

Let's start by deciding which judgments need our energy and attention.

In a world full of armchair experts, it's easy to get lost in what other people think, and I find it helpful to make a clear distinction between opinions that can influence me and those that can't.

Let's Grow!

Because my relationship with my children is one of the most important resources in their developmental process, I see it as my job to ensure that our connection remains intact and that intruders are not allowed to mess with that sacred circle of trust. This perimeter doesn't have to be openly discussed with everyone around us either. We all have different cultural relationships with elders and hierarchies, and we may need to break cycles covertly rather than openly announcing our departures from tradition.

But it is our job to prioritize our children's needs over other people's discomfort or opinions.

While I'm *very* invested in helping my children learn appropriate social behavior and awareness of others, I'm also determined that they know I'll be there for them when they need my support, even if that makes other people feel uncomfortable.

Who Gets Influencer Status with Me?

Growth in this area doesn't mean that we never listen to other people's insights about us or our children. It means we must make sure those insights are helpful and don't distract us from prioritizing our children's actual needs. If we spend energy trying to make everyone around us happy with our parenting, we inevitably neglect our relationships with our children. One way to evaluate whether those insights are helpful is to review who you give influencer status to. For example, people who get access to my heart and mind, especially around the topic of my children and my parenting, have to have the following core qualities:

1. Kindness: they are relationally focused and able to hold other people in their minds with understanding and compassion.
2. Curiosity: they have a capacity for wonder and learning.
3. Integrity: they live with consistent values and ethics.
4. Experience: they have lived a significant life or have labored significantly over scientific data.
5. Humility: they can acknowledge their own humanity and flubs.

6 Cultural competency: they are aware of how our different identities can affect each of us and can hold space for cultural differences between us while offering feedback or advice.

This list helps me weed out a ton of the noise, and it keeps me open to learning new things and hearing important feedback from the people who have earned a position as an influencer in my life. We all need protections in place so that we are not inundated and disoriented by the opinions of the 5 trillion people on the internet and in the grocery store who all think they have the right to tell us how to parent.

The Stranger Observer

This may be the easiest piece of advice to give on this topic. If you don't know someone and they're judging your children or your parenting, you don't need to do a darn thing. Ignore them. You have no idea who they are and cannot possibly assess whether they meet the standards to influence you. So default to no. They do not.

If someone is giving you a nasty turned-up-nose vibe while your child melts down in the ice cream aisle, simply imagine that they're dealing with some incredibly painful gas, and the sour look on their face is a result of serious indigestion. Quickly turn your back or switch aisles, and internally wish them well on their quest to release some good farts in their car on the way home.

If they make the bold (and intrusive) move to approach and say something judgmental or unhelpful, feel free to do whatever it takes to make them go away. Let them know that you're currently experiencing bowel distress and are close to pooping your pants. Or politely thank them for their advice, and then turn back to your child and continue the work you were doing to stay calm and focused on helping them regulate.

Trusty Tidbit

CHOOSING WHO WE LOSE

Change can feel scary, not just for us but also for the people around us. Especially for the people who raised us and who find reassurance that they did the right thing when we repeat their patterns.

Remember that loss of approval from the generation above us is a natural byproduct of a decision to break cycles on behalf of the generation we are raising.

When we work to heal and change, we incidentally shed light on the unhealed issues of other people in our lives, potentially making our relationships with them more tenuous. Nedra Tawwab says it perfectly: "A side effect of growth is losing people who liked you better when you were without boundaries or engaged in behavior similar to theirs.

Facing adversity, critique, and loss can all be a normal part of dealing with our sh*t. It doesn't mean we are failing or doing it wrong. We may lose the approval of our parents when we decide to use different parenting tools with our children than they used with us. We may lose closeness with a group of friends when we choose to address a drinking problem. Even though these realities can be painful, I believe they are losses worth facing when we know that we are giving our children what they need from us.

It is courageous and rewarding to put the well-being of our children above the discomfort of other people in our lives.

If you're dealing with virtual judgment from someone on the internet, I implore you to remember that people online are notorious for saying controversial things to get a rise out of you. Scroll on. Drink some water. Remember that if it doesn't feel helpful and aligned with your cycle-breaking goal, it's not worth your time. You do not need to defend yourself against the trolls. In fact the best defense against an online troll is disengagement. They can't get to you if you refuse to continue to walk over their comment bridges.

Whatever you do, don't devote a ton of emotional energy to conversations about parenting with random, judgy strangers. Your emotional energy is precious and limited. And the grocery store and internet trolls? They're seemingly infinite.

The Acquaintance

The situation gets a wee bit more complicated when the judgment is coming from someone who exists in our social orbit. It could be a neighbor, a teacher, a principal, or even a friend of a friend. Irrespective of who the acquaintance is, they exist in our world, making it harder to simply assume their judgy glare is bowel distress or to repel them with our own claims of gas.

But since we don't know this person well, they have still not hit influencer status in our lives. We don't have enough information to determine whether they are humble, kind, curious, ethical, experienced, or culturally competent.

This means we can choose our response. We can either decide to divest ourselves of this person sending real or imagined judgment our way, or we can do some investigative work and get to know them. For me, if it is just someone random that I don't need to deal with in my child's life, I cache them into the "can't care right now" bucket. I close the window to their potential judgments of me or my situation.

But if the acquaintance is someone who interacts with me and my child in an impactful way, I leave a window open a crack to get a sense of what they're blowing in my direction. This person could have some insights that I lack (this is especially important with educators because they see our children in a different context). Perhaps they hold information that will improve my understanding of my children or equip me with new tools.

However, this person's beliefs and values could also hinder my mission to give my children secure experiences with me. Or they might just want to "mean-girl" me. I need some time to figure that out.

It's a wait-and-see approach. I don't address my feelings directly with the acquaintance as we don't hold enough closeness to navigate my vulnerability yet. But I'm also not automatically shutting myself away from everything they have to say.

I then share these feelings with people I do trust and who are close to me—my certified influencers. My wise counsel can help keep me grounded while I shelve the acquaintance's potential judgments of me. Usually reassurance and support from the people who truly know me help relieve my concerns about the opinions of someone who is not close to me about my parenting.

The Concerned Loved One(s)

Now to the most complicated situation—when we feel judged by people who matter deeply to us.

If you are feeling judged by a loved one, first remember to use the list to check whether they're qualified to be an influencer in your parenting. Just because we love someone does not mean that we need to heed their advice.

If someone we love doesn't meet the criteria to influence our parenting, it's okay to listen to their concerns and smile and nod, but not dwell too much on their opinions. If what they say doesn't feel helpful in supporting you to become the parent you want to be, you don't have to spend lots of time and energy on it. Just move along, knowing that they have a different perspective that you don't align with.

If, however, the person sharing their concerns is someone whose influence matters to you, the first step in dealing with the situation is to admit to them that you're feeling judged. It doesn't need to be a confrontation, just a simple, *"I'm worried that you think I'm parenting the wrong way. Is that true?"* If this person really meets influencer status in your life, they will respond to your vulnerability with care and compassion. Perhaps they do have concerns they want to share with you, but they didn't know if you wanted to hear them.

The next step is about discernment. Listening to someone we love share concerns means hearing them out while continuing to listen to ourselves and our children.

In 2020, during the pandemic, I was knee-deep in twin babies and an extroverted five-year-old with no social outlets. Just like everyone else in the COVID shutdown, we were a hot mess, and my family started to feel concerned about my son's behavior. I caught wind of their concerns through the family-gossip-pipeline and also from their facial responses to situations that were causing my kid to melt down.

At the time, not everyone who was concerned met my criteria for influencer status. But some of my family members did, and a couple of others hit four out of five of the list's criteria, only lacking experience or expertise. So I gathered everyone together to discuss the fact that I was feeling judged (we were in a family COVID pod together).

Long story short, I was right. They had strong opinions on what they thought I should be doing differently with my son. They were concerned about him. Even though I felt uncomfortable with the conclusion they had reached—they thought I needed to be stricter when he was upset—their feedback helped me recognize that my son needed something from me that I hadn't figured out how to give him.

While listening to their perspectives on the situation, I realized that I had become less connected to my son after having my twin daughters in 2020. The two-baby-thing alongside the scary-global-pandemic-thing had led to me being less available for him than I'd been previously. His behavior was calling out to me not as a need for more harshness but as a need for more access to my heart and mind.

I melted down in tears and acknowledged with my family how overwhelmed I was feeling and how I'd become much terser and more stressed in my reactions to my son. They responded with care and concern, and it helped me recalibrate my approach to my relationship with my son.

It's been more than five years since that tense conversation, but its impact is still having positive effects on our lives. My family witnessed my vulnerable need for support, and I received their help in recognizing that I'd become out of sync with my son. We all learned a ton, and the concerns they had about my son have since vanished. He developed out of that stage/season, and I'm so thankful that *I heard my family's concerns* without *taking on all of their advice.*

Sometimes our loved ones have something to say that we need to hear completely, and sometimes it's just a part. Whatever happens it's important to assess whether the people giving us advice meet influencer status, and if they do, to filter through the advice and opinions they give us.

Opinions, advice, and perspectives from others are either going to help or hinder our growth. If someone genuinely wants to support us, they're not looking down on us; they're seeing us eye to eye and sharing their truths with love and understanding—even if it feels a little bumpy initially.

Is It Judgment? Or Is It Support?

Sometimes we might feel judged when someone is simply offering us support. This is important to recognize because if we view all feedback as judgment, we might miss out on some very valuable wisdom and information that could help us along our quest.

A few years back I noticed my good friend Matt was struggling with substance abuse. I had always sensed there was an issue for him around drugs and alcohol (hypervigilant child of a parent who struggles with alcoholism here), but the COVID lockdown and distancing measures had clearly exacerbated his problem.

His wife is also a close friend of mine, and she was calling me daily to vent about the frequency and volume of his alcohol and marijuana use. She was reaching a breaking point, and despite being in couples' counseling and sharing her concerns, her husband was only able to hear her pleas as judgments instead of invitations. Their marriage was hanging by a thread.

Later on in the pandemic, we were socializing in their backyard with all of our kids during the middle of the day, and he was clearly on drugs. I felt sad and worried about him, and more profoundly, sad and worried for his young kiddos.

I really didn't want to say anything to my friend because I knew there was a risk he would think I was judging him instead of trying to support him. But I knew he needed help. I also knew that I met my own criteria as an influencer.

So I wrote him a letter expressing my concerns about his relationship to drugs and alcohol and then helped his wife and friends write letters of their own. I showed up at his house with all of our letters, and when he saw me show up unannounced, he joked, "I smell an intervention coming on . . ." We sat on his couch and cried together as I read through each of the compassionately written notes from the most important people in his life. He definitely had to wrestle with feeling judged, but then he did something truly incredible. He asked himself, "Are these people trying to hurt or to help me?" And then he did something even more incredible—he sought out more help.

Matt is now years into a recovery journey and in graduate school to become a substance abuse counselor. His relationship with his wife and kids is thriving. It's been truly incredible to witness him grow and uncover all the parts of him that were buried under the drugs and alcohol he had been using to cope.

Sometimes we *feel* judged, but it's only because *we are judging ourselves*, and the leap is to start trusting that other people aren't looking down on us but are looking forward on our behalf.

Feeling judged is part of every parent's journey. So be selective about whose judgments you spend time and energy on, and keep your eyes peeled for the possibility that you aren't actually being judged; you're just feeling that way in the moment.

And always remember that you never know if someone is really being judgy, or simply regretting that gas station hot dog they ate for lunch.

Compassionate Self-Talk Scripts

- *"Not everyone in the world deserves to be on my influencer team. I can decide whose opinion gets ongoing access to my thoughts and energy."*
- *"No one knows my children and me as well as I do. I can trust myself even when other people don't."*
- *"I care so much about being a good parent that sometimes I think people are judging me when they're really just offering me help for the journey."*

Trusty Tidbit

REPEAT THIS PARENTING MANTRA

My life is not a show. My parenting is not a performance. The only judgments that matter are the ones that bring me closer to my kids and make me more confident in my mission to be a good enough parent.

Further Reading

Emotional Agility: Get Unstuck, Embrace Change, and Thrive in Work and Life by Susan David
How to Be You by Jeffrey Marsh
The Let Them Theory by Mel Robbins
Parenting in Public by Donna Haig Friedman
The First Rule of Mastery: Stop Worrying About What People Think of You by Michael Gervais, PhD, and Kevin Lake

How to Deal with Feeling Lonely

"Family isn't always blood, it's the people in your life who want you in theirs: the ones who accept you for who you are, the ones who would do anything to see you smile and who love you no matter what."

—DR. MAYA ANGELOU, MAYA ANGELOU'S OFFICIAL INSTAGRAM

We all feel lonely at times. We can feel lonely when we're actually alone, but we can also feel lonely when we're surrounded by people. Loneliness is the foreboding sense that we don't have people to rely on or people we belong with. It's a vulnerable and sometimes scary feeling. But like so many other sensations we face in our bodies, it exists to support our well-being. When we can effectively deal with our loneliness, it helps guide us toward greater investment in our relationships and social health.

How Our Loneliness Affects Our Children

Our children can usually sense when we're feeling lonely. They notice that we're feeling unsupported and disconnected from other people. I like to say that loneliness has a fragrance—they smell it even if we don't talk about it.

If the smell of loneliness comes in faint whiffs, the effect on our children is only to humanize us a little. But if the smell lingers for a long time or is especially pungent, it can have a more profound impact.

If we're feeling lonely and we're not trying to alleviate that feeling by reaching out to other adults in our lives, our children can feel pressured to try to meet our social-emotional needs themselves. This makes it hard for us to give them gift #1 of feeling that we can handle what they feel. This is a problem because it means they'll forsake their own social and emotional needs to try to comfort us and help us feel that we matter and belong.

While it might feel good at first to have our children notice our loneliness and try to reassure us, it's a big burden for a kid to carry. A burden that makes it harder for them to explore the world without looking back to check on us.

The other problem our loneliness can create for our children is that it can become a model they learn to emulate. Our lack of connection, or drive to form connections, can become the vision they have for their social worlds. Our children need to witness us connecting with people so they recognize the healthy pattern of building close and secure relationships.

Feeling lonely motivates me to connect more with the people in my life whom I trust to care for me when I'm vulnerable. I let people know that I'm feeling isolated and then ask directly for what I need. It could just be a quick text reassuring me that I'm not the only one struggling with a particular issue. Or it might be getting together to do something fun or to talk about a concern that's on my mind.

I never *want* to reach for help when I'm feeling lonely because the shame gremlins are usually running wild in my brain and telling me that I'm lonely because I'm weird or abnormal or in some way difficult to love. I usually want to feel sorry for myself and scroll the internet for proof that other people are getting together, and I'm on the outside of it all. But it turns out that doesn't make me feel better!

I've learned to always ignore the gremlins. They do not pass the influencer vibe (see page 68) check at all. Instead I try to remember all the times that people have told me that they really want to be there for me if I ever need them.

Let's Grow!

Loneliness stinks. But that doesn't mean addressing loneliness feels easy or intuitive. Especially if we've been lonely for a long time. We can feel so comfortable in our loneliness that it seems preferable to the work it would take to un-lonely ourselves. But if we want to give our kids the five gifts of a secure parent, then we have to deal with our loneliness. When we stir up the courage to step out of isolation, we relieve our children of the incredible burden of meeting our social and belonging needs. Then our children can focus less on being there for us, and more on growing into themselves.

When Our Loneliness Is Asking Us to Move the Furniture Around

Sometimes our loneliness is a *priority problem.* We're pouring ourselves into our work, our children, or our tendency to get lost scrolling through social media, and we're not taking time to prioritize the relationships in our lives that help us feel connected.

If this is the issue, only a small shift is required. We *have* people we belong with and can rely on; we just haven't been putting in enough effort to feel connected in those relationships. The solution to feeling lonely is to rearrange the "furniture in our living room" so that we place our relationships more centrally in the room.

As a parent with little spare time, I find it helpful to make "connection routines" with my friends and family. One group of my female friends commits to dinner every two months. Another group gets together for a week every year. I spend time with my brother and his kids every weekend. And Sunday night is game night with my immediate family. By prioritizing routine connection time, I can protect it more easily.

This modeling is so important for our children because it helps them learn to prioritize togetherness as part of their life rhythm. And given what we know about the impact of our relationships on our longevity and well-being, this lesson is one they truly need us to model.

When Our Loneliness Is Asking for a Whole Remodel

Sometimes we *don't have* people we can reach out to. We don't have relationships with people who are warm, safe, reliable and capable of cultivating belonging for us.

This type of isolation can happen for many reasons. As a result of internal factors, such as not believing we're worthy of quality close relationships or having trauma that makes it scary to get close to people. Or it can be caused by external factors, such as being geographically isolated from people who know us well or living in an area where we feel culturally isolated from people who share our identity or values.

No matter what internal or external factors have led us to this level of isolation, we and our children deserve our efforts to remedy the situation and to increase our relational support.

Our loneliness is asking us to remodel our people patterns when:

- We have no one to call to help us process tender emotions or tricky life situations.

- We have no belonging or group identity outside of our relationships with our children.
- We don't regularly spend time with any other adults.
- We have no one who knows our daily rhythms, thoughts, and needs.
- We rely only on ourselves and our own resources and don't reach for others in moments of celebration or struggle.

As social creatures we need other people in our lives to help us thrive. We need people to listen to us, show us empathy, give us advice and guidance, and most of all, help us enjoy our lives through play and belonging. Without those things in our lives, our bodies and minds enter higher levels of stress and discombobulation.

If we're not experiencing good relational care and community in our lives, it becomes a much harder challenge to give our children good relational care. Partly because we burn out faster, but also because our children can sense our isolation, and they intuitively know that it's not a good sign of well-being.

If we don't have our own social support, our children might sacrifice their social development to care for us. Instead of spending time with their friends or interests, they worry that we won't cope without them. This gets in the way of being able to go out and explore the world in the ways they need to for their continued growth and development.

Our children need to know that we're sturdy and reliable so they can launch off of us into the exciting task of exploring the greater world around them. If we're wobbly in our own well-being, it can make it harder for them to go as far as they're capable of in their own life adventures. That can be as true when they're in kindergarten as when they're creating their own family lives as adults.

We don't want our children to be burdened with the task of addressing our loneliness; we want them to be free to learn and grow and deal with whatever their lives bring them.

How to Remodel Your Relational World

1. **Blueprints before building**
   Take the time to consider what type of people you crave in your life. It might be that you need particularly caring and thoughtful people, or perhaps you need fun people who bring silliness into your life. If you don't know where to start, finding a therapist to help you can be a way to both decrease your loneliness and to get support in figuring out the blueprint for your relational remodel.
2. **Demolitions may be necessary**
   Sometimes we have to tear down structures before we can build new ones. If there are people in your world who take up a ton of space but do little to alleviate your loneliness, you may need to tear down those walls before you can put up sturdier ones.
3. **Start small and slow**
   We don't need a trillion people to feel connected, just a few good pals to journey with us. One connection at a time is a good way to pull ourselves out of an isolation pit. Make it a goal to find one new friend and work on developing a close friendship with them over at least a year.
4. **Anticipate duds**
   Not every firecracker you buy is going to work. Sometimes things just don't work out. That doesn't mean you're broken or unworthy of connection; it just means it wasn't the right fit or

the right timing. When a relationship doesn't pan out, ask yourself if there's something to learn going forward. And if not, just chalk it up to "you win some, you lose some." Don't let it deter you from continuing your mission to address your isolation.

5 **Invest in people who can both give and receive**
When we're remodeling a house, it's wise to use materials of the highest possible quality. Why? Because they last longer, and we don't have to remodel again in the future because of inferior materials. For similar reasons, we want to invest in people who are capable of giving and receiving care because it means they have the skills for a longer investment in a relationship. And we need to make sure that we're those types of people too. Bonding comes from truly doing life together, which means putting in the effort to care for the other person and letting them in enough to make a difference in our lives with the care they bring to us.

We all experience loneliness. But if we're careful to take responsibility for those feelings and meet the needs that underlie them, our children won't be put in the position of feeling responsible for our social well-being. And we'll be less likely to place guilt or obligation on them that could obstruct their own social development.

Compassionate Self-Talk Scripts

- *"My loneliness is not a sign that something's wrong with me, it's a sign that I need more connection than I'm getting right now."*
- *"It's normal to feel lonely at times, even when I'm surrounded by people. Cultivating deep connections is hard work, and the right people are not always available."*

> ***Trusty Tidbit***
> **MAKE A CONNECTION PLAN**
>
> If your children are worried about your loneliness and isolation, develop a connection plan you can follow to take responsibility for your situation. For example:
>
> Monday—call Susie
> Tuesday—drop in to a water aerobics class at the gym
> Wednesday—join Toastmasters
> Thursday—call Dad
> Friday—lunch with Jeremy
>
> A connection a day helps keep depression at bay. And also helps keep our kids from neglecting their own needs to try to take care of ours.

- *"This loneliness I feel is a stage or a season, and it won't be forever. I can choose to take steps toward deepening the connections I already have with people or finding new people to bring into my life."*

Further Reading

Becoming Kin: An Indigenous Call to Unforgetting the Past and Reimagining Our Future by Patty Krawec
Choosing Family: A Memoir of Queer Motherhood and Black Resistance by Francesca T. Royster
Find Your People: Building Deep Community in a Lonely World by Jennie Allen
How We Show Up: Reclaiming Family, Friendship, and Community by Mia Birdsong
The Art of Community: Seven Principles for Belonging by Charles H. Vogl
The Art of Gathering: How We Meet and Why It Matters by Priya Parker

How to Deal with Feeling Powerless

"I am no longer accepting the things I cannot change. I am changing the things I cannot accept."
—ANGELA Y. DAVIS, UNKNOWN SOURCE

There are so many things in life that we have no control over. *So many things.* As a highly sensitive person, I have feelings of powerlessness at least once a day, but usually upward of ten grillion times. Sometimes the feelings visit me when I'm processing stories on the news about seemingly endless occurrences of horrific human rights tragedies. Sometimes they come when my minivan door refuses to close because it's angry at me for some unspoken reason.

None of us has power over everything. And most of us have power over less than we would like to believe. (Except maybe David Blaine? Have you seen what that guy can do?!) For the rest of us mortals, including our children, life is full of realities that are outside our influence, and this makes learning how to cope with feelings of powerlessness *essential.*

Feeling powerless is only a problem when we see it as a permanent condition. When we lose complete sight of the things we have power over for a significant period. I call this being under the "powerlessness fog."

The powerlessness fog obscures our view of the things we can change to affect our situation. Things such as our attitude, our responses to the situation, and our ability to reach out to others for support.

When we're in the fog, we can only see the things that we *cannot* change. And if we stay in the fog long enough, we come to believe that we *are* powerless. Over everything. End scene. Cue numbing habits (on page 208). We check out because we no longer believe that anything exists outside of the powerlessness fog.

Powerlessness can transform from a visiting feeling into a habitual coping skill. When that happens we lose our ability to use our other coping skills. Which means we also lose our ability to be a reliable haven for our children.

How Does a Powerlessness Fog Affect Our Children?

Very few things get in the way of human growth quite as much as feeling chronically and completely powerless.

When we're stuck in the fog, we disconnect from responsibility and hope—two things that our children absolutely need to see in us in order to learn for themselves. And for them to feel they can trust us to care for them in whatever complex life situations they're facing (mucking up gift #1).

If this happens, we're not able to offer our children a parent who is empowered and sturdy. Our children become deeply connected to our "deflatedness" instead, and the pain that comes with our perceived powerlessness. This usually leads them to try to help us by taking over the role of the parent.

They may hide their needs or feelings as a way to "protect" us from more pain or burden in our lives. They may become advocates for us in our other relationships and focus on trying to help us feel better by persuading other people to do things they think we want or need.

It's also possible that they'll get stuck in our fog alongside us. Because our internal models of the world are profoundly influential on our children, our powerlessness fog can become part of their self-view. Instead of recognizing the things they're empowered to do, they get stuck staring at the barriers in their paths.

Whether they're getting stuck in our fog or feeling responsible to parent us in ours, our children need a dedicated effort from us to learn to clear the fog enough to take hold of the things that are within our power to affect.

Stepping out of the Fog Doesn't Mean Pretending We're on Cloud Nine

Just because we're working to take hold of the things within our control doesn't mean we have to pretend that everything is fine. Usually when we're struggling with a powerlessness fog, it's because some truly awful and harrowing things have happened to us or to people we love.

It's painful to live in a world where life isn't fair, and it's even more painful when that unfairness has specifically targeted us. The barriers to safety and thriving are not equally distributed across all our obstacle courses.

Which is why processing the harm and inequity we have faced, or are facing, is a necessary part of clearing the powerlessness fog. We need to be able to process the unfairness of our lives so that we can help our children learn to process the unjust realities they encounter along their journeys. It's healthy to feel angry at those injustices, and it's important to experience whatever grief comes with them.

But that doesn't mean we should relinquish all the power we have over our lives. It means we acknowledge the abuses we've endured and then work vigilantly to claim our influence over the things we can change and create.

Holocaust survivor and psychiatrist Viktor Frankl says this perfectly in his book *Man's Search for Meaning* when he describes what he learned during captivity in four different concentration camps and eventually losing his entire family in the Nazi genocide: "Everything can be taken from a man but one thing: the last of the human freedoms—to choose one's attitude in any given set of circumstances, to choose one's own way."

Let's Grow!

Stepping out of a powerlessness fog doesn't mean we forget the obstacles on our path; it means we continue to claim our lives even when outside forces are trying to take them from us. The ultimate cure for feeling powerless is cultivating serenity. Serenity is the capacity to do these three things:

- Let go of what we don't have control over.
- Take action toward what we do have control over.
- Recognize the difference between those two things.

Serenity is a state of emotional sanity in the face of an often-insane world. It doesn't mean we think everything is hunky-dory; it means that we're clear about what we can do with the cards currently dealt to us. Here's a step-by-step guide to how we create serenity in response to feeling powerless:

Step One: Acknowledge the Pain That Brought the Powerlessness Fog In

Yes there are almost certainly some big, bad things that have happened, or are happening, to us that brought the initial fog. What are they? And what do they mean to us?

Write it in a journal, tell it to friends, make sure your pain feels acknowledged and understood by both you and the people you trust.

Sometimes acknowledging this type of pain means stomping your feet like a toddler while you scream profanities up at the sky. Other times it means crying and slobbering onto the sleeve of someone close to you. Or it might mean writing your story and putting its painful truth down on a page. Do whatever it is that helps you understand, feel, and release the pain of the things you cannot control.

Step Two: Go on a "What Can I Control" Scavenger Hunt

Once we've released the pain about the things outside of our control, we can move on to seeking out the things we *can* do in our particular situation.

Make it a game. Find each of these things to win the scavenger hunt:

- A drawer in your house that can be cleaned out and better used
- A favorite book you can't remember all the way through that you can read again
- A favorite TV show you haven't watched in a decade
- A memory of a time someone else was truly kind to you
- A memory of a time you were truly kind to someone else
- A new recipe that you've never cooked before (or if you're kitchen-challenged, a new restaurant you've never tried)

- A sentence that describes what you hope people feel in your presence
- An inspiring quote from a book or the internet
- Something in your closet that feels comforting to wear (blankets count)
- Something in your home that smells good to you
- Something you can do with your breath when you are feeling powerless (hint: it could be holding your breath, making it deep, or learning a breathing trick like square breathing)

Add to this list and ask other people to improve it for you as well. There are *always* places of hope to scavenge even in the deepest powerlessness fogs.

Find the Hands and Handles

Powerlessness makes our heads droopy and keeps our eyes glued to the floor. We can't see a way out because we're more focused on the bottom of the pit than the openings that exist above it.

This is normal. It's hard to look up when the sky feels so foggy and heavy. But if you look up long enough and with enough determination, you'll find there are people outside of your hole willing to help you climb out.

Look for the hands reaching down toward you. The hands might be coming from someone close to you or someone you don't yet know well. Whoever is saying, "Are you okay? Is there a way I can help?" is the owner of the hands I'm talking about.

If you can't see any hands, it might simply be that people don't realize you're feeling stuck under a fog. Call up to them directly and ask them to help you get a ladder: "I'm not okay, and I'm not sure how to get out of here. Can you help me?" They might know how to give you what you need, or they might help you find people who can.

Grab hold of whatever you can to fight for your right to live in the sun again. In addition to human support, there are other handles we can use to help us feel our power. Sometimes it involves getting a prescription from our doctors to help our brains reset with some added serotonin absorption (antidepressants have been a helpful part of my journey when I've been stuck under a thick and seemingly unmovable fog). Sometimes it means taking advantage of the support we usually reject out of fear of burdening people. The steps we take to actively shift out of feeling powerless are cures for the feelings of powerlessness.

This is because as we start to take action, our brains and hearts will sense that there are places where we do hold agency. We're not all powerful, but nor are we ever completely void of the ability to impact our situation.

Compassionate Self-Talk Scripts

- *"I was not in control of what happened to me, or even how my body and mind instinctively responded to it. But I'm now in control of how I choose to process it and care for myself moving forward."*
- *"It was disorienting to experience the abuse or trauma I went through and to be powerless over a moment or a particular situation, but that does not mean I'm entirely powerless; I always have my ability to decide to heal."*
- *"I got stuck and forgot there are things I can do. I don't need to beat myself up for that, I just need to keep looking forward so that I can unstick and move forward differently."*

Trusty Tidbit

DO A POWER PUMP-UP

When we're struggling to get our heads out of the powerlessness fog, we can help ourselves and our children by doing a "little bitty power pump-up." It's an effective way to help clear the fog by doing small and accomplishable tasks that can help our brains notice that there are things under our control. Here is my routine for getting myself boosted out of the fog:

- Make my bed
- Feed my cats
- Read one small poem by Mary Oliver or Rupi Kaur
- Clean out my wallet
- Organize a drawer or closet
- Write a kind text or note to someone I care about

Even though these efforts and their impacts are small, they remind me that even in the worst circumstances, there are always things that I can influence.

Further Reading

Embodied Activism: Engaging the Body to Cultivate Liberation, Justice, and Authentic Connection by Rae Johnson, PhD
Essential Labor: Mothering as Social Change by Angela Garbes
Man's Search for Meaning by Viktor E. Frankl
Revolutionary Mothering: Love on the Front Lines, edited by Alexis Pauline Gumbs, China Martens, and Mai'a Williams
The Enneagram for Black Liberation: Return to Who You Are Beneath the Armor You Carry by Chichi Agorom
The Mountain Is You: Transforming Self-Sabotage into Self-Mastery by Brianna Weist
Volume Control by Jen Butler

How to Deal with Feeling Regretful

"Failure is not falling down, but refusing to get up."
—TRADITIONAL PROVERB OF UNCERTAIN ORIGIN

My husband likes to remind me that just as our children are in a developmental process, *so are we* as parents. None of us can come to this journey fully equipped with *all* the knowledge and resources we need for every possible scenario we will face. No one has ever been us before, and no one has ever been our particular children before. And no one has faced the chemistry that exists between us and our children at this particular point in human history.

So it makes sense that we make mistakes along this journey. Without a full map of what lies ahead, we all take wrong turns or end up going the exact opposite direction of our intended destination. Hence, feeling regretful.

It happens.

When we realize we've swerved off course, our regret comes bumbling into the room at full volume ("I wish I hadn't taken that dumb shortcut!!!" or "Why didn't I just keep going instead of turning around??"). Seeing things with time and perspective can help us understand where we went wrong and what we could have done differently that we didn't see at the time.

Even though we all inevitably feel some regret along our parenting journey, it doesn't mean we know how to deal with those feelings. And if we aren't careful, regret can become an emotional quicksand, spiraling us into anxiety, depression, and overcorrections that we regret later on.

How Do Our Regretful Feelings Affect Our Children?

Well it depends! When we feel regret over something we've said or done (or not said or not done), and we use that regret as a motivator to repair our relationships with our kids, our regret benefits them.

Losing our minds over our children's missteps is something that 99 percent of us do at one time or another. Did I once threaten to give away one of our cats after one of my children covered her head to toe in blackberry ice cream? Yes. Did I make that threat knowing fully that this particular child of mine has soul-mated for life with this particular cat? Yes. Yes I did. And when her face fell with the deepest of agonizing grief and betrayal, did I regret my desperate attempt to teach her a lesson by using this particular empty threat? Of course I did. I regretted the desperate and cruel threat I made to try to teach her about cat ice cream boundaries.

Which led me to work on apologizing. It was important for her to feel my regret because it helped her understand that I knew my choice had hurt her and was far below the line of emotional maturity I try to offer my children.

But if I let myself dwell in that regret, its helpfulness could have easily worn off—even by the next day. When we allow ourselves to soak in regret we can get visited by the powerlessness fog (see page 86) and lose sight of what we can do to move forward (getting in the way of gift #1, showing we can handle what they feel, and gift #2, showing we can understand their perspectives).

Chronic regret appears more selfish than selfless. If we remain staring in the mirror at our flaws, we can't turn around to face the people who are in the room with us. Our kids need us to feel appropriate regret, move toward repair, and then move out of the regret before it transforms into deadly quicksand, taking us out of the present and future before us.

Let's Grow!

Regret is a history teacher. Its primary area of expertise is the past, but as a result, it does have some nuggets of wisdom to help us build a better future. We all know that history tends to repeat itself, but it's less likely to do so if we take the time to understand exactly why something went wrong and what can be done differently next time.

When we notice that we're feeling regretful about something in our parenting journey, it's important that we pause and study the lesson we're presented with. *And* that we do so with a learner's heart and don't weaponize our past mistakes against our present selves.

Study Don't Sink

The best way to prepare for a regret study is to remind ourselves of these three things:

1. We did the best we could with whatever information, support, or mental state we had at the time.
2. It takes maturity and courage to acknowledge regretful feelings. The first step toward growth and change is always to be honest with ourselves about the hard stuff.

3. There's a difference between seeing a past choice as a negative thing (regret/guilt) and seeing it as proof that we are a negative thing (shame/identity). "I made a mistake when I did *X*, *Y*, or *Z*" is a far more productive way to study regret than, "The fact that I did *X*, *Y*, or *Z* is proof that I'm a terrible parent and person." Ditch the shame—it isn't true and it won't help you or your child to heal.

When we feel regret, we're learning about what happened in the past so we can take different actions to help us have a more connected future. Healthy regret is about looking back long enough to look ahead with hope, not dwelling in self-condemnation or flagellation.

Lay Out the Lessons

When we're feeling regretful, there's usually a web of lessons all tangled together. I find it helpful to untangle the web by asking myself these questions:

1. What is the thing I regret doing or not doing?
2. Why do I regret it? (What was the impact on my children or my relationship with my children?)
3. What was the context I was living in at the time? (What was happening in my work, health, relationships, culture, and development?)
4. What was missing from that period in my life that would have helped me do better?
5. Have things changed in my life since then that have allowed me to understand this regret in a different way than I could at the time?
6. What have I already learned from this regret?
7. What do I need to do or learn to do to prevent this regret from happening again?

Forgive Yourself First

This may seem counterintuitive at first, but hang with me because it's a very important part of handling regretful feelings effectively. When we notice that we've done something that caused harm, suffering, or disconnection for our children, we're usually met with a serious dose of panic. It's truly disturbing to realize that we've done the opposite of what our core heart wants for our children. We want to be parents who act as safe havens and secure bases, and who can build our children up and help them fly to their fullest potential.

So when we recognize that we are responsible for pain or suffering for our children, it's heart-wrenching in a way that very few things in life can compare to.

If we move too fast to apologize to our children, we'll bring our panic energy along with us, making it much harder for them to trust our repair. Instead of our children being able to sense that our regret is about *their* pain, our pain will take over the moment.

How can we possibly forgive ourselves for hurting or neglecting our children? We remind ourselves that our children didn't stop needing us. We're still their parents, no matter what age they are, and to do better in the future, we have to find a way to see our past selves with compassion so we can get back to parenting. Moving forward isn't about erasing the hard stuff, but it's also not about making it our identity. It's about allowing ourselves permission to grieve.

It's sad to realize that we've not been able to give our children the full, secure experience we wanted them to have with us. It's good to let sadness out, to honor it by crying and sharing it with safe and wise people we know. When we allow the grief to release, it starts to live outside of our bodies instead of getting trapped in our hearts and becoming anxiety or bitterness.

We let it out so we can make room for the pain our children are holding from our past missteps. If we don't release our pain and make room for theirs, we're setting up for a new regret in the future. You deserve to feel free from this pain in the same way that your children do.

Make Amends

Once we've grieved and forgiven ourselves for our missteps, we can begin the process of effectively making amends with our children.

Sometimes the amends process is short and simple. Sometimes it's a marathon. But the starting line is the same: checking in with our child about what they feel ready for. This can be done in whatever communication style your child prefers—a written note, a text, an email, or even a conversation over coffee. Here's an example script for a check-in:

Parent: "*Hey, I've been thinking about x (how I handled our fight last week, how much I worked when you were younger, the way I responded to your anger when you were growing up, etc.), and I want to apologize and hear more about how it impacted you. Do you feel up for that anytime soon? If yes, would you rather we talk in person or write letters back and forth? Or send telegrams? (I'll have to figure out how!) I want this to be about you getting what you need, so I'm good with whatever timeline and preference you have.*"

If the regret is about something small or recent and you sense that trust was not disrupted in your relationship with your child, making amends can be as simple as knocking on the door and saying, "*I want to apologize for being so harsh earlier about the spilled cereal. I really scolded you, and you didn't deserve that. Accidents happen, and my crustiness was about other things. I'm sorry I took it out on you.*"

Sometimes our children receive our amends easily and even enthusiastically. They feel relieved to have something acknowledged and to get back in sync with us. At other times they mistrust the amends or are plagued by other stressors in their present lives and lack the energy to process the past. No matter how they respond, it's our job to continue working to understand the impact of our actions or inactions, grieve the things we cannot change from the past, and work to build a healthier and more secure future.

Feelings of regret are supposed to guide us toward feeling forgiven and forward-facing. If we find ourselves continually looking back at the past, we often miss the road right in front of us. Let the regret do its thing by revealing the lessons that need learning, but then let the regret transform into deepened compassion and hope toward the person you are now and the person you're growing into.

Compassionate Self-Talk Scripts

- *"Just because I regret something doesn't mean I can't learn from it and do better in the future."*
- *"I did the best I could with what I knew at the time. Now that I know more, I can do better in the future."*
- *"My regrets show me how much I care about my children and about being the type of parent they can rely on. Every thoughtful parent has some regrets."*
- *"Regret is not a place to land and stay, it's a train to take toward greater understanding and forward learning."*

Trusty Tidbit

BOXING UP UNHELPFUL REGRETS

1. Find two medium-sized shoe boxes.
2. Label the first box: "Things I wish I had done differently."
3. Label the second box: "Things I've learned from my mistakes."
4. Whenever you have a regret, write it out and put it into the first box. If you can let it go and forget about it without guilt or worry, that's great—you've accepted your regret. If, on the other hand, you're struggling with the regret, take it out of the box and write on the back of the paper all the lessons you've learned as a result of getting something wrong. Then, once you can tell you've truly learned from that regret, place it in the second box and make a vow to yourself to fully let it go. You've learned from it, and that's all a regret is asking from us so we can lay it to rest. Take a deep breath and be super proud of yourself that you have two boxes. You're not just someone who gets things wrong—you're someone who learns from the things you get wrong.

Further Reading

Get Over It: Overcome Regret, Disappointment, and Past Mistakes by Dr. Liisa Kyle

Matters of the Heart: Healing Your Relationship with Yourself and Those You Love by Thema Bryant

Self-Compassion: The Proven Power of Being Kind to Yourself by Kristin Neff, PhD

The Power of Regret: How Looking Backward Moves Us Forward by Daniel H. Pink

How to Deal with Feeling Rejected by Our Children

"The fear of being rejected becomes the fear of not being good enough."
—DON MIGUEL RUIZ, *The Four Agreements*

It can be straight-up agonizing when our kids don't want to return our affection, trust in our advice, or, heaven forbid, be seen in public with us. Plus feeling rejected can easily send us spiraling down into a pit of toxic shame feelings (see page 129).

I've been there, and so has every other parent I've ever met. It's a normal part of a parent-child relationship.

Big R Rejection vs Little r Rejection

I'd like to clarify for all of us the difference between big *R* rejection and little *r* rejection.

Big *R* rejection is the very painful experience of someone wanting *nothing* to do with us, exiting fully from our lives. Our children only big *R* reject us if they choose to go no-contact with us after they leave our homes. Children only go no-contact with parents if there's a *significant negative situation* at hand. It could be a repeated history of neglect or abuse, an external force in their lives pulling them away from us (such as a cult dynamic or abusive partner), or it could be a symptom of a severe mental illness, such as schizophrenia or substance abuse, that affects our children's ability to feel safe in the world, even with us.

STOP

Big *R* rejection, when our children stop having contact with us, is incredibly painful and complex. This level of rejection requires professional support and guidance. Because there are so many possible variables at play, when this happens to us, we need people to help us process the situation and guide us toward the next best steps in our unique dynamics. For free resources and additional support, head to estrangement.com to get connected to community and professionals who specialize in this tender situation. Alternatively see How to Get Yourself to Therapy on page 265 for additional resources.

Little r Rejection

The most common forms of rejection we feel from our children are the more subtle refusals and dismissals they make toward our attempts to connect with them:

- It's dancing in the car and being met with a face of horror instead of joy.
- It's giving a gift to our children, only to find out that their preferences changed yesterday, and they don't want it.
- It's approaching them with open arms when they've hurt themselves, only to have them yell in our faces and run into the arms of someone else (even if that person is their other parent, it still stings).
- It's offering them advice or insight and watching them ignore or rebuff our attempts to help.
- It's rejecting aspects of our heritage, culture, way of life, or religion (in subtle or not-so-subtle ways).

Little *r* rejection might be best reframed as "how our children let us know that what we're offering isn't in line with what they either want or need." It isn't a parenting fail, or even something to feel deeply worried about, but it can certainly trigger deep-seated concerns about ourselves and the status of our relationships.

How Does Our Feeling Rejected by Our Children Affect Our Children?

It depends on what we do in response to the feeling.

If we react too strongly to those feelings and proclaim them to our children ("Why don't you want to spend time with me today? Don't you love me anymore?"), we'll certainly rattle them with panicky guilt toward themselves or deepening alienation from us, and we'll compromise gift #2, our children feeling that we understand their perspective.

If we tease them or make light of their communication with us about what they want or don't want, they could feel misunderstood or devalued by us, messing up gift #3, for them to be able to feel how much we want a close relationship with them.

However, if we can see these little *r* rejections as communications about their needs and preferences and get curious about them, we can transform them into deeper connections with our children.

Let's Grow!

Let's break down little *r* rejections into categories to understand how to respond effectively when they arise.

Rejection of Emotional Support

One of the greatest gifts (and the greatest expenditures of energy) as a parent is the honor of soothing our children when they're upset. The instinct for our children to run into our arms when they're tender or distressed is the foundation of our bonding and belonging together. But that doesn't mean we're guaranteed they'll always choose us as their safe haven.

Children tend to have a hierarchy of preferences when it comes to soothing their needs, so when multiple parents or caregivers are present, there tends to be a top choice. In my house this is usually me, partly because of the role I played in carrying and birthing my children.

My husband is an incredible nurturer—he's loving and open and gives empathy and responsiveness when my children are in pain. In my absence they run into his arms without any hesitation. But he tells me he often feels rejected when I'm there. He wants to be able to soothe them and hold them when they're in pain, but instead he feels like they see him as an obstacle to getting into my arms. This is attachment preference at work and has nothing to do with the quality of the bond my children have with my husband.

Luckily if caregiver preference is the reason our children are rejecting our emotional support, they're still getting emotional support from us when those higher up in the preference order are absent. And this strong preference usually lessens as children mature and feel less flooded when feelings enter their bodies.

If you often feel rejected because your children choose someone else for emotional soothing, it's important to empathize with and validate their preference ("You really want to be with your mom/dad/grandma right now, and that's totally okay").

The more our children sense that we're not threatened by their desire to be held by another caregiver, the more they start to associate our presence with soothing. If we can remain calm and accepting of their preference, it communicates to them that we can handle their other emotions.

If, however, we sense that our child is rejecting our attempts to soothe them even when we're *alone* with them, it's probably one of two scenarios:

One: The emotion they're feeling is anger. Anger is an emotional state that tends to seek *space* instead of *soothing*. When we're angry we're more sensitive to finding touch overstimulating or intrusive. If our children run away from us when they're upset about a boundary, or they're flooded with such a huge surge of emotions that they feel disoriented, it probably means that they need a low-stimulation environment for a moment to regulate (alone in their room, post door slamming).

When this happens:

1. Let your child relocate the storm to another room (or under a couch).
2. Wait one to three minutes for the storm to settle.
3. Walk *slowly* toward the storm.
4. Use a gentle voice or a note on the outside of the door or room to say something supportive and empathetic like, "*I can sense you're feeling overwhelmed, and I'm here to hug you or hear you out whenever you feel ready. Take as long as you need.*"
5. Wait a few more minutes if you're met with silence or rebuke.
6. Try again.
7. Repeat these steps until the storm has changed into a tender rain of tears or a willingness to be held or heard.

Two: We need to work on our soothing responses. It might be that our children are not getting the responses they need from us to find our presence soothing. In other words, it might be an "us" problem. Maybe we didn't get emotional support as children, so we lean in too intensely and smother them with our anxiety when they're in pain. Or it could be that we do the opposite and come across as dismissive or disinterested in their pain. If the issue is our responses, then we have attachment-related work to do—see the Further Reading in this chapter for help with that.

Quality Time Rejection

Another common form of little *r* rejection that we experience from our children is a rejection of quality time with us, which is often due to differing interests. Perhaps we invite them to cook with us, but they have no interest in culinary pursuits, so they make an excuse and head elsewhere. They rejected the context for the quality time, but not necessarily the quality time itself.

Then the solution is fairly simple—we convert our attempts at quality time into things that fill our children's bucket. If they like to craft, we craft with them; if they want to throw a ball around, we get sporty.

We can still ask them to help us cook dinner, but not with the illusion that they'll be excited about it. Cooking dinner might be a skill we want them to learn, but it won't be a situation in which quality time ensues.

Quality time rejection also naturally decreases as our children age and develop more independence and interest in their peers. Especially around adolescence, the contexts that would have previously translated to enthusiastic quality time no longer have the same hold. They're focused on building bonds with their friends instead.

One of the most frequent pieces of advice I hear from respected parents of teens is to recognize that we're no longer in charge of deciding *when* quality time occurs. Our teens are. Which means that it may happen late at night when they come home from socializing.

All we can do is say "yes" to as many opportunities as they give us, knowing that they don't come as frequently as they used to. (I think of this as parenting whiplash—we go from being asked to play with them every seven seconds to only being offered quality time with them every seven weeks.)

As someone who loves the experience of adventurous eating, I naturally want my children to develop the same passion. I have visions of my family all over the world, happily huddled around tables full of unique cuisines. You might imagine your children playing a sport you love or feeling passionate about the same faith traditions. It's natural to want our children to love the things we love.

While it's natural for us to want to share the things that are sacred and meaningful to us, it's also normal for our children to have their own separate experiences of those things.

We have to find a way to offer our children opportunities to experience the things we love without creating pressure for them to feel exactly as we do. I've found the following guiding principles very helpful in maximizing the likelihood that my children will try new things with me and enjoy quality time together in a variance of arenas.

Nudging Over Pushing

Sometimes our children will oppose something initially because they need more exposure to it to discover the joy it brings. For instance, an eight-year-old might not want to learn how to play chess but could develop into an adult who loves it.

We can't know for sure whether our children *really* don't like something or whether they just need time to develop a taste for it. So when offering opportunities to my children, I find it helpful to ask myself, "Am I nudging or pushing?"

Nudging:

- Offering opportunities to try something (inviting them to play chess with us)
- Singing the praises of something I love (talking about how excited I am to play chess with my friends)
- Enjoying the thing I love around my child (playing chess with other people around my child)

Pushing:

- Requiring my child to do the thing I love even when it brings great distress ("You will play chess with me or you will not get to see your friends this weekend!")
- Using fear or shame tactics to try to gain interest ("You're going to feel embarrassed when you are older and are the only person who doesn't know how to play chess")
- Teasing or badgering our children for not liking what we like

When we take a nudge approach to something we love, our children will often grow to love it too. If we stay away from the temptation to push, then at least there's no chance of causing a rift in our relationship. Perhaps they never grow to like playing chess, but if that's the worst thing that happens, then we're both pretty lucky.

Invitations Over Mandates

When we want our children to learn to love something, it's helpful to imagine that we're inviting them to a celebration. When I eat food that I love, my mouth celebrates. When I play board games that I love, my brain celebrates. When I play volleyball (court only, not sand or grass), my whole body celebrates.

What's the most effective way to encourage someone to join us in something we enjoy? Well it's certainly not by telling them they have to. (Trust me, I've tried this and continue to test it, especially in moments when I am overtired or stressed out!)

The most effective way to introduce our children to something we love is by confidently inviting them to our party.

When I'm cooking food, especially food that's new to my children, I start by cooking it for myself and showcasing my enthusiasm for it. While their enthusiasm for certain foods doesn't always match mine, they're far more willing to try it, and sometimes it hits the taste bud jackpot.

Remember that enthusiasm and joy for things we love are incredibly persuasive teachers.

Acceptance Over Pressure

When our children give us a solid *"No"* in response to an invitation, it can hurt our feelings or incite panic in us. We're experiencing loss, even if it's micro-loss for a moment. Perhaps we made a delicious dinner with all of our children's preferences in mind, but as we place it on the table, noses curl up and disgust groans commence in unison. The shared dinner we envisioned is lost. Instead of joy and gratitude, we're faced with culinary rejection.

What we do in response to that grief is important.

The first thing is to be kind to ourselves in response to our disappointment. It's totally legitimate to be sad when our kids can't join in our joy. I usually say something to myself like, "Well that wasn't how I saw this going. I was really looking forward to enjoying this meal together, but I can see that's not going to happen tonight."

By accepting that we're sad, we're more likely to be able to accept our children's feelings, including their gag response to our beautiful meal. If we can remain accepting of what our children are feeling, they often put their guards down and ease a little toward willingness to try something new.

For-Now Feelings Over Forever Identity

When we're sharing something we love, we're often sharing a part of ourselves.

The things we love can become part of our identities and how we connect with other people, which is why it can feel so threatening when our children don't feel the same way as us about something.

But when we start ascribing an identity to our children based on a potential temporary feeling or preference, we can be limiting their future choices.

For example, I noticed one of my daughters was sticking her tongue out at her plate and pushing her mushrooms away from her other food at dinnertime. I said, "It looks like you don't want to eat the mushrooms tonight, that's okay." Her whole body relaxed.

When the following month her sister went on a mushroom bender, my daughter caught her sister's enthusiasm and asked for a bowl full of them for lunch one day, all because we hadn't labeled her as "someone who doesn't like mushrooms." Did she finish them like her sister? No. But she told me she enjoyed them that day. When our kids are still developing, it's helpful to frame their preferences as momentary feelings and not markers of who they are or who they will become.

Affiliation Rejection

Our children will reach an age when they start to shift their feelings of belonging beyond our family walls. They begin to value their peer relationships at a different level than they did when they were little.

This can be as small as wanting to sit by their friends at an event instead of with their family. Or it can be big, such as choosing to bind their lives and loyalties to someone else by making a marriage commitment.

It's important not to view their nuanced changes in identity as a rejection of their belonging with us. They don't have to choose. They can love being with their friends and still hold their places in our families. This is so important because if we take it personally or hold a grudge, they'll slowly relinquish their places in our lives. If we make them choose, they're unlikely to choose us. Why? Because it's the way our species propagates and continues the cycle of life.

Our children need to go forth and live beyond our homes so that some of them can reproduce and keep the human race moving forward. Even if they don't start their own families, their instinct will still push them out into the world and propel their ongoing development.

Trusty Tidbit
REFRAME AND REASSURE

When our kids little *r* reject us, it's helpful to label their behavior in a way that reminds us that it's not big *R* rejection and then reassure them that it's okay for them to do what they need to do (even if they're still learning how to do it maturely).

- If my kids ask me not to hug or kiss them, I say, "I'm so glad you know that you have affection autonomy and get to say what you don't want to do, even with me."
- If my kids say "no" to hanging out with me, I reply, "I'm so glad that you know what you need right now, even if it is different from what I wanted from you."
- If my kids want comfort from someone else, I say, "I love that you have multiple people who show up for you and that you can choose the support of who you need in this particular moment."

Even if your children are too young to understand these complex topics, these statements help us to regulate and repel any instinct to overreact to the situation.

Compassionate Self-Talk Scripts

- *"It makes me feel sad when my children want someone else to comfort them, but it doesn't mean that they're big-R rejecting me."*
- *"I wish my child loved the same things as me, but since that's not the case right now, I can learn to love the things they do and keep inviting them to what I love, hoping that one day it grows on them."*

- *"My children are complex and unique individuals, and it makes sense that sometimes they want or need things that I can't give them. I can at least give them acceptance of that reality."*
- *"Everyday rejections are part of every relationship, just as every day connections are. It's okay if my children and I go in and out of sync with each other as long as I stay generally available, accepting, and warm."*

Further Reading

Adult Children of Emotionally Immature Parents: How to Heal from Distant, Rejecting, or Self-Involved Parents by Lindsay C. Gibson, PhD

Drama Free: A Guide to Managing Unhealthy Family Relationships by Nedra Glover Tawwab

I Never Thought of It That Way: How to Have Fearlessly Curious Conversations in Dangerously Divided Times by Monica Guzman

Learning to Disagree: The Surprising Path to Navigating Differences with Empathy and Respect by John Inazu

Raising Securely Attached Kids by Eli Harwood

Reconnecting with Your Estranged Adult Child: Practical Tips and Tools to Heal Your Relationship by Tina Gilbertson

Walking on Eggshells: Navigating the Delicate Relationship Between Adul Children and Parents by Jane Isay

How to Deal with Feeling

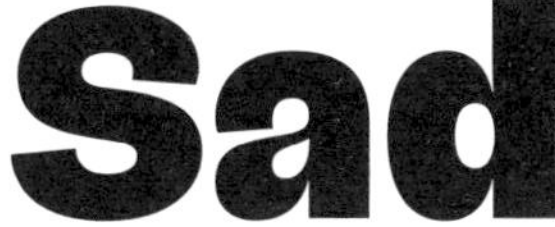

"Every one of us is losing something precious to us. Lost opportunities, lost possibilities, feelings we can never get back again. That's part of what it means to be alive."

—HARUKI MURAKAMI, *Kafka on the Shore*

It's common for people to want to avoid sadness at all costs, seeing it as a negative emotion or a sign of weakness. But me? I have a strange relationship with sadness. As a therapist, I think sadness is incredibly valuable. I witness the service that sadness brings to our lives as an integral part of the healing process.

There's a reason we use the phrase "I need to have a good cry." When we can feel our sadness and release it from our eyes, it acts as a medicine for our hearts. Especially when we do so in the presence of people who care about us. Sorrow helps cleanse our hearts, minds, and bodies of pain so that we're freer to be in the present and to hope for the future.

This is in contrast to despair. Despair is often mistaken for sadness, but they're actually wildly different. Despair is what happens when our pain mixes with hopelessness. Despair takes our pain and paints it into eternity. Despair tells us that the hurt we feel cannot be healed, while sadness tells us where it hurts so we can release the pain and open our hearts to the possibilities of the future.

Despair = stuckness
Sadness = movement

If we can honor the sad feelings that arise in our bodies, releasing them will actually make us feel *better*. But if we did not grow up in environments where the adults around us knew how to express and release sorrow, the process of learning how to do so ourselves can feel complicated.

How Does Our Sadness Affect Our Children?

It depends whether we're stuffing it away (avoidance), drowning ourselves in it (preoccupation), or releasing it with care (processing).

If we're stuffing our sad feelings away, our children learn that sadness is shameful or a burden to other people (compromising gift #1, feeling we can handle what they feel, and gift #4, feeling that we can show up for them when they need us). If they see us hide our pain, they'll assume it means that pain and tenderness are to be handled in isolation. If they don't have any other strong examples of how to respond to sadness, they'll be stuck with the same stuffing-away traditions that we inherited. ("If his sadness is not worthy of being seen, mine must need to be hidden too.")

On the other hand, if our sadness triggers us to sink into despair, it can overwhelm our children. If we get flooded with despair when we feel sad, they end up feeling scared for us and naturally question our ability to handle their tender or distressing needs. ("If she can't handle sadness in her own body, I definitely shouldn't overwhelm her with mine.")

I want our children to know that sadness can be felt and that they can trust us to support them through the sorrowful emotions they feel, big or small. ("My parents feel sad just like I do and will understand and know what to do when I'm feeling sad and need support.")

Let's Grow!

There's a common thing many of us do with sadness: we rank it according to size. This is especially common if we grew up in a home where there was little support for our tender emotional states. Instead of simply acknowledging sadness and letting it out, we assess whether we think the thing we're feeling sad about is big enough to deserve acknowledgment. We look at emotions other people are experiencing and say, "What they're going through is *really* sad, I shouldn't feel so sad about this small thing."

I think of this as the "Sadness Olympics." We only give permission to feel sadness that we think has earned the right to be on the podium. Things like death, wars, and famines. The big dogs of heartbreak. This leads us to dismiss our everyday sad feelings and stuff them down, ignore them, or find ways to numb them away.

Which, ironically, is a very sad way to live. Because when sadness becomes trapped inside our bodies, it transforms into numbness, disconnection, and even depression. While we may think we're honoring someone else's big sadness by ignoring our own, we're just obstructing our own needs for processing and connection.

And when we ignore our sad feelings, we miss opportunities for connection. Everyone knows what it feels like to get our hopes up only to be disappointed, or to miss someone close to us, or to wish for something that we can't have. Sadness is a thread of belonging.

When we courageously share sadness with others, we become emotionally lighter and closer to those people.

If you struggle with the Sadness Olympics, I want you to imagine that instead of the awards going for sadness severity levels, they are given for our ability to acknowledge, share, and release our sadness when it comes knocking. Even if it's about spilled milk. Whenever sorrow visits, it's asking to be acknowledged and let out.

Release the Sadness

The next time you feel sad, I want you to:

- Stop, give yourself a moment to pause from whatever you're doing, and simply feel the sad feelings in your body. (Tears will likely float up to your eyes if you have fully stopped.)
- Acknowledge the source of the sadness—what are you feeling sad about? Maybe you just had dinner with your extended family and you're sad because you feel politically polarized from one another. Maybe you were turned down for a job you really wanted, or maybe your favorite salsa has been discontinued (Territorial House salsa, I will never forget you).
- Divulge your sadness; in other words, share it with someone who will understand it or offer a caring response. Even if that someone has a tail and long whiskers. Sorrow is for sharing (remember sorrow and misery/despair are not the same thing!).

When we do this, our bodies will amplify the sad feelings enough to release them from our eyes. We cry, or at least tear up, which helps the sadness go outward instead of imploding inward.

Dealing with Olympic-Size Sadness

Although all of our sadness deserves our attention and care, the sorrow that accompanies big grief and loss is unique. While we don't all face exactly the same losses, we all face loss in some form throughout our lives.

We lose people we care about to death, miscarriage, divorce, changes in ideologies, or even sudden and unexpected moves or estrangement. We can also experience significant grief when we lose jobs, careers, or aspects of our health, and of course, when one of our furry or feathered friends meets the end of their journey here on earth.

When losses occur while we're raising our children, we face a very particular pickle. Not only do we have to deal with our own grief, but we're also responsible for supporting our children in working through theirs. While the road through grief and loss is always bumpy, here are some key things we can understand and do to help us get through it with as little additional fallout as possible.

Edit Expectations

When we lose someone we love, or something pivotal in our lives, our capacity is initially compromised. This is a hard pill to swallow because it means that when grief and loss initially visit, we not only lose the someone or something we are grieving, but we also lose our ability to function normally.

- Our ability to stay calm is reduced.
- Our ability to take care of ourselves and others is reduced.
- Our ability to be responsive to work, friends, or family is reduced.
- Our ability to feel hopeful or joyful is reduced.

When we're in the early stages of a loss (at least the first year), we're thrown off our center of gravity as we relearn how to walk on an entirely new planet. Knowing this doesn't make it less uncomfortable, but it can prevent us from beating ourselves up about changes we have no control over.

If we've lost our center of gravity, we can at least offer ourselves (and our kids and partners) the understanding that we won't be living life at the same pace or clarity that we were before the loss.

When we're in the throes of grief and loss, we won't be able to do all the same things we were doing before life punched us in the stomach. That does not mean we're failing; it means we're surviving, and that's truly something to be proud of in the midst of grief.

Feel the Feelings

If we're navigating grief and loss as parents, we can feel pressure to "be strong for our kids," which often gets translated into putting on a charade of being okay. But grief and loss need to be released. We need to cry our eyes out until we can see straight again.

This is most therapeutic if it's done in the presence or arms of someone who can hold our pain with us. If grief and loss have come into our lives, then the sorrow and ache they bring to our bodies have to be given space to be felt and released so that we can keep living even while we're processing who or what is gone.

Let the Village Help

Let them make you meals. Let them clean your car, pick up your kids, or do your grocery shopping. Whatever they're offering to do or whatever it is that you are struggling with, let the village help. Even if the village is a neighbor whom you didn't know well before. Grief is a great time to grow your village.

This is part of human nature: to be supported by our community. Can it feel awkward or uncomfortable? Sure. Especially in individualistic cultures. But the more you embrace help at this time, the richer your life will be. Hope doesn't revive in isolation; it revives when we realize that we don't have to suffer alone.

Mention the Messiness

Our kids can feel when we're in the throes of the big dogs of sadness. We're not operating in normal vibrations, and they sense we are going through something even if they don't know what it is. When we let kids sense the confusing changes in us without an explanation, they tend to think something is wrong with them or their feelings. Which is why it is so important to mention the messiness to make sure they know that what they're sensing is real, and it's not their fault or their responsibility.

My son was two and a half years old when I had my first miscarriage and three when I had my second. Pregnancy is obvious on me—I throw up every single day and resort to living exclusively on cinnamon raisin bread. Instead of leaving him confused, we let him know each time we were expecting. That meant he knew each time our expectations were crushed by the grief of knowing that the baby we were hoping for didn't make it into our arms.

He could sense that we were sad, so we shared truthfully with him so he could at least understand why the sadness was with us. And it was with us for a while. We went through two losses, a surgery (my uterus got a remodel), countless tests, unsuccessful fertility treatments, and finally a successful IVF pregnancy that gave us our incredible daughters, but of course, did not replace the losses we experienced or the time that passed in between.

When we're going through loss, it's important to mention it to people who care about us and to tell our children an age appropriate truth about the situation so they know the name of the thing they can feel emanating from us.

Losses Upon Losses

One of my close friends, Heather, went through a season of extreme loss while she was in the middle of parenting a toddler. She had multiple miscarriages, as well as losing her second daughter, Blakely, at week thirty-nine of pregnancy—a devastating, life-altering loss.

The loss in itself was excruciating, but it did something big losses often do, it uncovered losses from the past. The pain of losing Blakely made it impossible for Heather to keep ignoring memories of childhood sexual abuse that she had been running from for so many years.

Confronting the family abuse was a deeply painful process that cascaded into even more loss. She had to end her relationship with an unrepentant abuser, and to add salt to the wound, she had to face the loss of relationships of other family members who did not believe her. Heather didn't only lose pregnancies and her daughter Blakely, she lost her ability to deny trauma, and in doing so, she lost people who wanted her to stay in denial.

Through an inspiring determination to grow and heal, and with the support of courageous friends and caring therapists, she came out the other side of this grief cyclone with her sense of hope still intact. The she funneled her pain into her determination to support other people who have survived child loss or childhood sexual abuse. When I asked her how she did that, this is what she said:

> By allowing the anger, the sadness, the disappointment, and the grief to seep through every part of my bones. I have learned that loss is one of life's greatest teachers.
>
> When we are in the throes of loss, we need people to spend time listening to us while we try to accept things that never fully make sense.
>
> We need to let people help us with the mundane daily tasks that become inherently overwhelming.
>
> And most of all we need people who learn to see us as changed but continue to love us just the same.

Big loss triggers big truths.

When we are in the throes of loss, we learn things about ourselves, our past, our present, and the people around us.

We need help healing. We need help staying away from the bitterness quicksand. We need help believing in the kind of care and treatment we all deserve from our loved ones.

And most of all, we need help learning to be ourselves in a world that has changed profoundly around us. I recently saw a quote that resonated: "My parents may not understand my healing, but my children will."

There's safety in being understood by others who've walked a similar path.

While our stories are unique to us, there's comfort in knowing we're not alone.

Connecting with a local support group of other loss families helped my husband and me feel seen and understood. Hearing other people who had survived sexual abuse and were brave enough to stand up and say "no more" also encouraged me to keep fighting and reclaim that part of my story.

Loss has shaped me, but ultimately it has made me clearer on what matters and who I want to be, teaching me that healing is a journey best shared with others.

Sharing Our Sadness with Our Kids

Our children learn how to use utensils by watching us. They learn how to form words into sentences by listening to us. They learn how to feel and how to respond to their feelings by watching us respond to our own emotional cycles.

We can help our children trust us with their feelings by showing them we're capable of feeling our emotions and managing our responses to them. This means not shutting them off at one end of the spectrum and not drowning in them at the other.

That being said, letting our children see us feel our emotions is not the same thing as *asking our children to help us understand or alleviate our emotions*. When we share our sadness with or around our children, we need to be careful not to:

- Dive into despair or catastrophic thinking
- Ask for them to be in charge of reassuring us or helping us heal
- Share graphic or mature details about something they can't understand
- Ask them to take our side in a divorce or conflict situation
- Lay heavy uncertainties on them

It's totally okay for our children to see and know that we feel sad about something. As long as we also communicate that our role with them is still the parent, and that we're actively receiving the care and support we need from other adults in our lives while we're caught up in that sadness.

Movies vs News vs Our Lives

My children regularly see me express sorrow when something sad happens to the characters in a movie. I'm a crier. I feel things deeply, even when the things are made up and on a screen. But I find that my ability to feel sorrow for fictional characters normalizes feelings of sadness for my kids. And since my response is to something fictitious, it's usually pretty safe to say that the emotions won't overwhelm my children or lead them to feel responsible for my emotional state.

I also let my children experience my sadness when I'm processing sad things that are happening in the world outside of our community. But I'm more cautious about what and when I share because my heartbreak over real-world tragedies is heavier than the tear juice I drop over Anna and Elsa's parents getting lost at sea in the movie *Frozen.*

It's hard for me, even as a grownup, to emotionally process the reality of wars, natural disasters, human rights violations, or even smaller-scale individual tragedies that often make the news. When we're processing the big nightmares of the world, we have to be particularly thoughtful about how we filter down the information into something age-appropriate.

STOP

If you're feeling so sad or down that it feels impossible to imagine life getting better, you may be struggling with depression. Please reach out to a friend or health care professional whom you trust to get care asap. If you're seriously considering self-harm or suicide, please immediately contact 911 (or whatever emergency number is used in your location) and ask for help in getting support to stay safe.

Here's how that could sound:

Kid: *Mommy, are you crying?*

Parent: *Yes, honey, I just learned about something on the news that made me feel sad.*

Kid: *What happened?*

Parent: *Some people were really hurtful to some other people.* Or *some people lost their lives.*

Kid: *What happened?*

Parent: *You'll learn about things like this when you are older, but this story is too heavy to put into your heart right now. It's too much for someone your age. But it is something that people my age are working to fix, so I'm going to work out what I can do to help the hurting people, and I'll let you know if I can find a way that you can be a part of that help too.*

The other time to share our sorrow with our children is when we're navigating something sad in our personal lives. A few years ago we lost my husband's grandmother, Jean, and his Aunt Janis (who had been a special person in my life since I was fifteen years old) during the same holiday season. Grandma Jean was in her nineties and ready to pass. But Aunt Janis was in her mid-sixties, and we all felt the deep tragedy of her life being cut short.

When I went with my son to say goodbye to Grandma Jean in the hospital, I cried openly as I told her how much I loved her and how much I was going to miss her. As I let my tears flow, my son was able to connect to his own tears. He was also sad about facing a final goodbye with his great-grandmother. When we left the hospital room and headed to the car, we held hands and cried together as we discussed how strange and baffling life and death felt in that moment.

I did not, however, share with him about some of the more complicated feelings that were mixed up in my tears. Disagreements about worldviews that Grandma Jean and I had experienced over the years, or my fear that our extended family might become less connected after losing Janis, who was very much the heart glue that kept us all connected. Those complex elements of my grief would have been too much for my seven-year-old to process.

But he absolutely needed to see me feel and express my sadness to normalize the expression of the feelings that come from losing people we love. Because the grief of losing people never fully goes away. Grief is a regular visitor knocking on the doors of our hearts, reminding us of the things and people we have loved but lost. When it shows up, we cry, hug, and then feel the relief that comes with being sad in each other's arms. Sadness deepens our bonds when we can swim the seas of sorrow together.

Checklist for Sharing Our Sadness with Our Kids

- ☐ Let our children witness that we feel sad feelings and can handle them.
- ☐ Model self-compassion toward ourselves when in tender emotional states.
- ☐ Contain and process feelings of despair with other adults, not our children.
- ☐ Edit our disclosures to information that will not overwhelm our children or lead them to feel adult-level responsibilities or pressure to "take our side" in our personal conflicts with other adults in their lives.

Compassionate Self-Talk Scripts

- *"Sadness is my body's way of helping me heal from losses and pain."*
- *"It's okay to cry in front of my children to model for them that it's okay to cry."*
- *"My sadness connects me to other people and helps me build community."*
- *"Sorrow can feel big at times and small at other times. This is normal and not something I'm doing wrong."*
- *"No matter what is making me feel sad, my sadness is valid and deserves to be understood and expressed so that it can be released from my body."*

Trusty Tidbit

SADNESS AND LOSS GROW US

Write this profound quote on a piece of paper, cross-stitch it onto a pillow, or paint it onto a canvas and display it somewhere you will see it every day:

> *"When nothing softens the grief, may the grief soften me."*
>
> —ANDREA GIBSON

The things that grow from our losses are truly miraculous and can offer us a place to sit and remember who or what we have lost, and to see what it is that we're now becoming without them.

Further Reading

Bearing the Unbearable: Love, Loss, and the Heartbreaking Path of Grief by Dr. Joanne Cacciatore, PhD

Furiously Happy: A Funny Book About Horrible Things by Jenny Lawson

It's OK That You're Not OK: Meeting Grief and Loss in a Culture That Doesn't Understand by Megan Devine

The Noonday Demon by Andrew Solomon

Notes on Grief by Chimamanda Ngozi Adichie

When Things Fall Apart by Pema Chödrön

You Better Be Lightning by Andrea Gibson

How to Deal with Feeling Shame

> *"I define shame as the intensely painful feeling or experience of believing that we are flawed and therefore unworthy of love and belonging—something we've experienced, done, or failed to do makes us unworthy of connection. I don't believe shame is helpful or productive. In fact, I think shame is much more likely to be the source of destructive, hurtful behavior than the solution or cure. I think the fear of disconnection can make us dangerous."*
>
> —DR. BRENÉ BROWN, *Daring Greatly*

Shame is an incredibly uncomfortable set of sensations that rushes through our bodies when we feel we're bad. Not that we *did something bad*, but that we *are* bad. "I messed up when I yelled at my kids" is very different from "I yelled at my kids, which proves that I *am* messed up." Shame is a feeling that hijacks our humanity and blurs our perspective on our worthiness for connection. It makes us want to hide our vulnerable parts away from other people.

This is especially tricky on our parenting journeys. If we're stuck in shame, we're more likely to check out, blow up, or splatter the shame onto the people closest to us in the form of contempt. And we're less likely to remain confident and connected.

Unlike some of the other feelings we experience, shame does not have an adaptive gift to give us. Shame does not help us do better. It just leads us to feeling desperate or hopeless.

How Does Our Shame Affect Our Children?

Shame distances us from our children. When we're whirling inside of a shame storm that's sending us cruel messages like "you're a terrible parent" or "you're stupid and useless," we're faced with a primal panic that pushes us into a pit of despair. This mucks up gift #3, our children sensing that we want to be close to them.

If we feel that we *are* the terribleness that we're feeling, our instincts to hide and numb become pronounced. We lose our ability to see ourselves and our situation with nuance and accuracy. This is scary for our children because they rely on us and adore us.

But there's a big difference between small incidents of shame that we address quickly and prolonged shame states.

Before my sweet mama was able to get the counseling and psychiatric support she needed, her unresolved trauma often spun her into prolonged shame cyclones. I remember as a child witnessing the cyclones enter her body and take over her sense of self. It felt like she was being kidnapped by an invisible army of intruders who were attacking her from the inside. When she was in a shame spiral, I couldn't access the mom I needed, wanted, and trusted.

My dad's relationship with shame was more subtle, but more constant. I could feel it in his defensiveness anytime he had to be reminded about something he forgot, and certainly in his relationship with alcohol. He kept the shame intruders groggy and incapacitated by lulling them with a few drinks every night.

Watching my parents get stuck in shame broke my heart as a child and made it harder for me to focus on just being a kid. It made it darn near impossible for them to give me gift #1. I didn't think they could handle what I felt, so I held in my most tender feelings and either shut them down or shared them with other people.

I don't blame my parents for getting stuck in shame. I know they were navigating their own childhood traumas and neglect. But I do grieve those years that were covered in shame intruders, and believe that so much could have been different for all of us if there had been clear resources available to help them fight shame at the source.

As parents, it's our job to fight off shame intruders so that our children have emotional access to us.

Let's Grow!

The good news is that shame is never the truth. Shame is a distortion of something we're processing or experiencing. Any shame voice or sensation in our bodies that's condemning us, belittling us, or is harsh or cruel toward us is a false messenger. Whenever those things arise in us, here are some key ways to approach them:

Clean Up on Aisle Shame

1 **Identify What Spilled**
When we're saddled with an unwelcome visit from shame, the first step to dealing with it is to put the feelings into words. We can do this in our heads or on paper, but our brains need us to separate the feelings from the facts. The feelings tell us that we should find a cave to hide in and never come out again. The facts tell us what triggered the feelings of shame in our bodies. Example: "When I realized I forgot about my daughter's basketball game, I was flooded with shame and the idea that I was a bad parent."

2 **Ask Someone for a Mop**

Call up or reach out to someone you trust to hold your story with kindness and understanding. Tell them what happened and what you felt, and then ask directly for them to help you reject the shame from your experience. Research has shown that the more we share our shame with others, the less we feel it and the less power it has over us.

Example: "Can you help me to believe that I'm still a good parent even though I flubbed?"

3 **Mop Up the Shame**

Allowing ourselves to trust in the reassurance of people we're close to can temper the sense of isolation that shame triggers inside us. When we bring our shame to someone safe and caring, we discover that they don't want to banish us to a cave for eternity, which helps render the shame messages null and void.

NOTES ON CHRONIC SHAME

For some of us shame is not a visitor that comes and goes, but a resident that has rooted itself deep into our identities. This is usually because we grew up in shame-ridden families in which no one knew how to clean up the mess on aisle shame. Our family was covered in it, and no one could escape its sticky residue.

Or we experienced sexual abuse or bullying that eroded our connection to our dignity.

This is not simply shame, it's unresolved trauma.

If you feel constantly unworthy and nothing seems to help, check out the section on feeling traumatized on page 142.

Trusty Tidbit

MEANINGFUL MANTRA

Repeat after me (and repeat to your children):

Nobody is ever unworthy of love and connection.

Yet everybody experiences feeling unworthy from time to time.

Being unworthy is a myth; feeling unworthy is a pesky reality we all face.

The best way to face it is to share it openly with each other, since we all know what it feels like.

Compassionate Self-Talk Scripts

- *"Just because I made a mistake, doesn't mean that I am a mistake."*
- *"The only way out of past mistakes is through understanding, compassion, and care."*
- *"If I wouldn't want someone to talk to my kid with condemnation, then I can work not to talk to myself that way."*
- *"There is no parent on earth who doesn't have sh*t to work through, and the best parents on earth are the ones who are willing to try."*

Further Reading

The Unshaming Way: A Compassionate Guide to Dismantling Shame by David Bedrick

Transform Your Guilt and Shame: Evidence-Based Strategies to Heal from Trauma and Adversity by Carolyn B. Allard, PhD, ABPP

You Are Your Best Thing: Vulnerability, Shame Resilience, and the Black Experience by Tarana Burke and Brené Brown

Daring Greatly by Brene Brown

How to Deal with Feeling Stressed

"Stress is the most common and unifying experience we have as human beings."

—DR. ADITI NERURKAR, *The 5 Resets*

Life inevitably comes with stress, but being a parent quadruples the size of the stress load that we face. Not only do we have to contend with trying to keep ourselves alive, dressed, and fed, but we have to do it for our children too! *Daily!* And all while trying to figure out where in the hades we last put our phone and our keys.

With perfect timing, I'm currently feeling stressed as I'm writing about feeling stressed! My children and I took turns getting strep last week and through the weekend. Which means that everyone also took turns waking me up in the middle of the night every night, staying home from school, and needing my care and attention on a minute-by-minute basis. Even though I cherish the fact that I get to take care of my children when they're sick, it's also physically and emotionally draining. And it's impossible to stay on top of anything else.

And just as I was sitting down to try to steal an hour to catch up on life, I received an email from an employee of my publisher asking me to provide some details for a proposal. But it turned out that the email wasn't actually from my publisher. It was from a shady crime syndicate in Russia. And their deceptive phishing scam duped me into entering my email and password before I realized what was happening.

Now I'm behind on life *and* may also be losing my identity to a crafty criminal approximately 5,233 miles away from me. (Don't worry, I changed all my passwords!) I also have only twenty minutes until I need to pick up my son from the bus stop and head into the weekend, when my to-do list will continue to mock me without any further opportunity to reduce it.

The good news for me, and for you, is that while we don't get to decide whether or not we face stressful situations in life (curse you, internet pirates!!!), we *can* learn effective ways to respond to the stressful feelings that life creates inside us. The goal is to model for our children what it looks like to handle our stress instead of letting our stress handle us.

We have a stress mess if:

- We're chronically preoccupied with our to-do lists and responsibilities.
- We stay in constant motion and believe that we can never rest.
- We're chronically cranky and annoyed.
- We struggle to have fun or to be goofy or playful.
- We prickle easily and feel on edge most days.
- We relate to the people we love as tasks to be completed.

How Does Our Stress Mess Affect Our Children?

When we live in a *chronic* or *intense* state of stress response, we're no doubt exposing our children to increased stress. They can see it in our clenched jaws, our frenetic movements, our constant managing and shuffling, and our inability to be present and calm.

Depending on our children's temperaments, they might feel responsible for trying to reduce our stress (entering into a parent role), or they may start to avoid us and put distance between us.

The difference between a stress mess and a managed stress isn't necessarily less stress (so many of the stressful variables in our lives are out of our control); it's about finding a regulated response to stressful feelings.

Let's Grow!

These five steps for responding to stress are rooted in research and have been tremendously helpful to me in my personal growth journey, and also for my clients, friends, and family in theirs.

Step One: Expect Some Stress

I find that many parents have an unrealistic expectation of themselves to be permanently serene and calm. This is not a real thing. Nor is it what our children need in order to feel secure in their relationships with us.

They need to see that when we feel stressed, we take the necessary steps to manage our responses to the stress and don't (usually) overreact to it. The best way to demonstrate this is to anticipate that these stressful feelings will be a regular part of our lives.

This doesn't mean we expect to be stressed all the time but that stress is a feeling that will show up regularly in the life of a human parent. You're going to feel stressed. So am I. We're in this together.

Step Two: Evaluate the Stress Source

Stress can come from external sources, including internet phishing pirates, or it can come from internal sources, such as the delusional expectation that I can efficiently tackle my to-do list during the cold and flu season.

When stressful feelings arise, it's helpful to determine whether we need to take external action (change your password immediately Eli!!!) or adjust an internal belief or expectation. What I'm doing with my internal stress right now is reminding myself that no one will lose their life or limb if our laundry pile is unfolded for the next couple of days. And that the people who are texting me know how many children I have and how much I'm juggling. If it takes another week to reply, our friendships won't be beyond repair.

If our stress is external, the best way to handle it is to take an action step toward addressing that issue. We might send a quick text letting someone know it's going to be a few days before we can respond properly, or cancel a plan that can be rescheduled. It doesn't mean our stress will disappear, but it can reduce. And it will keep us from getting deeper into the stress cycle.

If my stress is internal, I find the most helpful way to curb it is to call friends who can help me adjust my beliefs or expectations. I have a group of friends called "The Still Got it Gals" who regularly chat on an app called Marco Polo (it's basically Snapchat for old folks), and they regularly give me input on my internal areas of stress to help me let go of unnecessary internal pressures.

Step Three: Externalize the Stress

One of the most common traps stress feelings can lock us into is believing that stress is a part of our identity ("I *am* stressed"). There's a funny thing that happens when we say we *are our feelings*. Rather than having more influence over them, they take over us. I call this "internalizing our feelings."

We should "externalize" our feelings instead by labeling them as something outside of ourselves. Instead of "I *am* stressed," which implies that we've become one with our stress, I say, "I am *feeling* stressed," which makes the stress a visitor in my body. One that comes with a message but doesn't have to spend the night.

Then I take it further and write out on a piece of paper, "I'm feeling stressed about . . ." and I write whatever is causing the tension in my body. I find that when I fill that blank in with specifics, even if it's with a list of seventeen different issues, I feel some of the tension release. It helps me see that the things I'm stressed about live outside of my body and can be addressed over time, even if not immediately.

Step Four: Experience the Sensations

Stress comes with physical sensations. Most people describe stress as an increase in tension throughout their bodies. Some of us feel it in our shoulders, some in our hips, some in our jawlines, and some even in our hands and feet. Wherever the sensations of stress play out in our bodies, they make it challenging to relax.

When we notice that stress tension is present in our bodies, the first step to releasing that tension is to let ourselves feel it. When we take a mindful moment to pay attention to the physical tension, it helps our brains to release it. It signals to us that we're safe enough to stop and observe.

It can be helpful to do a tension scan by starting at the tops of our heads and simply noticing where our bodies feel tight or constricted. When we notice an area of tension, we can focus on that particular spot and work to relax those muscles. By doing this all over our bodies, we can reduce our physical stress. And by changing our body sensations, we can enter a calmer state of mind.

I've become so good at this practice that I can guide my clients through it, and my kids too. Our stressful feelings live in muscle tension, so this is an incredibly powerful hack for reducing the volume of our stress.

A NOTE ON SYSTEMIC STRESS

Some of the stress we face comes from navigating unfair treatment or policies from the systems we live under. Systemic stressors affect us differently depending on our identities and our access to resources and support.

If we're experiencing stress from systemic injustice, we're dealing with stressors that can only be relieved fully through systemic change. Which is something we can work toward but don't have full control over.

Even if we can't eliminate the stress that comes from systemic realities in our lives, we can seek out support from others who are familiar with the same stressors. When we process our systemic inequity encounters with people who understand our experiences, the solidarity we gain can buffer the impact the stress has on our bodies and hearts.

Step Five: Expedite the Stress Cycle

When tension is active inside our bodies, it needs a release. Here are a few practical ways we can help our bodies release the tension:

1. Crying—when we cry we're releasing tension from our bodies via our tears and the heaving that can accompany a good cry.
2. Active exercise—moving our bodies increases the feelings of constriction, which then helps us experience a greater release when we stop moving.
3. Stretching or yoga—slow, mindful movements while focusing on breathing and intentional poses can also help release stress. This doesn't have to be in a studio or for a whole hour, just a few minutes a day to help our bodies release and relax.

4. Grunting, growling, or yelling—obviously this one needs to be done where the people around us won't worry that we've gone totally feral (and no yelling *at* other people). But when we allow ourselves to express guttural noises of frustration, it helps move the stress from our bodies into the air around us. My favorite is a good howl.
5. Sexy time—if you're someone who enjoys sexual connection and release, this is a free way to help your body process stress. (Please note that this is not a reason to pressure someone else into sex. There is *no* situation in which your partner ever owes you sexy time. Sex is a gift that must be wrapped in consent. If your partner isn't interested, take care of yourself!)

We all live with varying degrees of stress and different levels of resources to help us deal with our stress. If you're a single parent with a low income and no family support, your ongoing stress will be significantly higher than someone with generational wealth and an actively supportive family.

Remember that none of us can be stress-free parents, but we can become more competent at completing the stress cycle by using the resources available to us and by being kind to ourselves when resources are scant and our stress is understandably high.

Compassionate Self-Talk Scripts

- *"I deserve care and rest even when the to-do list never gets done."*
- *"Stress is part of life, but I can take steps for myself or get help from my community to improve how I cope with it."*
- *"Even when I'm faced with automatic stress responses in my nervous system, I can choose how I react to the stressful responses."*

Trusty Tidbit

SEEING WHAT OUR KIDS SEE ABOUT OUR STRESS MESS

The next time you feel caught in a stress mess, ask your kids for their expertise. They study you and have a good idea of things you might be able to change about your responses to your life stressors.

Ask them, "Do you have any feedback you want to give me on how you think I could handle things around here to reduce the stress?"

Kids are smart. They might tell us about the worries we can let go of more often or the things we're doing that are making it harder on ourselves. They might even offer to chip in and help with something if we follow up with, "Do you think there are any tasks you could help with to reduce the stress mess this week?"

Stress is best shared and divided, not kept on one person's shoulders. Our children are meant to help carry the practical tasks of our household, not the emotional task of trying to regulate our responses to stress.

Further Reading

Burnout: The Secret to Unlocking the Stress Cycle by Emily Nagoski, PhD, and Amelia Nagoski, DMA

How to Keep House While Drowning: A Gentle Approach to Cleaning and Organizing by K.C. Davis

The 5 Resets: Rewire Your Brain and Body for Less Stress and More Resilience by Dr. Aditi Nerurkar

How to Deal with Feeling Traumatized

"Trauma is not what happens to you but what happens inside you."
—**GABOR MATÉ**, *The Myth of Normal: Trauma, Illness and Healing in a Toxic Culture*

I feel so grateful to be parenting in a time when trauma has been well researched, understood, and made mentionable. We know a lot of things about how trauma affects our bodies, minds, and lives, and what recovery from trauma can look like. But even with so much information available to us, it's still fundamentally complex to understand and deal with. Let's start by understanding it.

There are three aspects to trauma:

1. The traumatic *experience*: any event that threatens our sense of safety, dignity, or belonging
2. The traumatic *response*: the bodily sensations that are activated within our nervous systems to help protect us during the traumatic event
3. The traumatic *narrative*: the story we tell ourselves about what happened to us both externally and internally

To describe those aspects in even simpler terms: *trauma is made up of the things that happen to us, the things that then happen inside of us, and the meaning we make out of those first two experiences.*

Let's say a large grizzly bear enters a grocery store when we're in the produce aisle choosing some navel oranges. We look up and see him heading in our direction. We would be having a *traumatic experience* because a grizzly bear running toward us in any context is a threat to our sense of safety.

As a result of our safety being threatened, our nervous systems would activate a fight (throw oranges at the bear), flight (run!!!), freeze (play dead), or faint response (become unconscious so we're not awake for whatever might happen next) in an attempt to protect us from harm. This is our body's *traumatic response.* Traumatic experiences activate physical sensations in our bodies, such as our hearts beating more quickly, our sight becoming blurry, our muscles constricting so we can rapidly run or hide, or our stomachs getting woozy right before we pass out (thank you, vagus nerve!).

If we survive this bear-meets-produce traumatic event, then the third part of trauma takes place: *the meaning we make out of what happened.* We might conclude that we were brave and leave the experience feeling more equipped for future grizzly bear run-ins (a positive post-traumatic self-narrative). This positive conclusion would reduce the trauma response in our bodies, shortening the amount of time we're feeling traumatized.

Or we might conclude that we were stupid to leave our house that morning and blame ourselves for believing it was safe to go to the grocery store (a negative post-traumatic self-narrative). We might conclude, "I'm not safe anywhere," which increases our traumatic response and keeps it on a loop. We now feel traumatized when we leave the house to go anywhere.

The way we internally narrate a traumatic experience and response has a profound impact on whether or not that trauma gets resolved or gets stuck on a loop replaying inside our minds and bodies.

The first two elements of a trauma, experiencing the event and the responses our bodies have to the event, are out of our control. We don't get to decide whether a bear invades our local grocery store, and we can't decide whether we run and hide or fall unconscious next to the blueberries. Traumatic experiences and responses don't give us time to make decisions. They are things that happen to us.

But after we've survived a traumatic experience, we do have some control over how we write the narrative about what happened to us and inside us. Even if we initially come face-to-face with a negative post-traumatic self-narrative ("I'm a weakling and didn't dare to fight the bear"), we can edit the story to offer ourselves recovery and healing. We can pause and recognize that, unless they have large weapons, human beings don't win battles against bears. And oranges don't count. Our body made a wise decision when it fled, froze, or fainted. Our body knew that our best chance for survival was not hand-to-paw combat.

How Do Our Encounters with Trauma Affect Our Children?

It's all about the narratives that follow the trauma. If we're stuck in a negative post-traumatic self-narrative, then our traumatic feelings have a big impact on our relationships with our children. Trauma that hasn't been fully processed prevents us from being emotionally attuned and available. This gets in the way of gift #1, our kids feeling that we can handle their feelings.

Instead of offering an emotional haven, our nervous systems set off alarm bells in confusing ways that can disorient our children in the world and reduce their instinct to seek regulating support from us.

If, on the other hand, we put in the work to write a positive post trauma narrative about ourselves, then our children actually gain an advantage from us. Because if we've completed healing work on our trauma feelings, then our children will understand that what doesn't kill you really does make you stronger. Not to mention the fact that people who have healed from hard things also become more compassionate, connected, and creative.

Let's Grow!

The best way to write a positive self-narrative after a traumatic experience is with the support and witness of caring people.

Write and Share the Story of What Happened to You, and an Impact Statement

This advice comes straight from a therapeutic approach called "Cognitive Processing Therapy." When we write and share our trauma narratives, it helps our minds and bodies make more sense of them. And when we write out a statement about the impact the trauma has had on our lives, it helps us to separate ourselves from the things that have happened to us. This is achieved most effectively with professional support, especially when our traumas are complex, but it can also be a powerful healing experience to share with the people in our "real" lives.

Although it can feel uncomfortable to talk about traumatic events, it's when we tell our trauma story to people who see us as worthy of care and understanding that the disturbance we feel about the events decreases. Others can help us notice the details in the story that may not be initially clear to us as we acknowledge and release the scary and shame-inducing ideas that are haunting us.

Edit Out the Shame and Guilt Cousins

We want to look for unhelpful shame and inaccurate guilt that keep us locked in trauma states even after the event has ended. Editing out shame and guilt changes how we see ourselves, which helps our brains understand that we're no longer in the traumatic situation. We need friends, therapists, or other community supports to say, "It seems like you reacted really quickly, and that kept you alive. I'm so glad you didn't try to fight the bear and end up dead!" See How to Deal with Feeling Shame (page 129) for more on this.

Let the Feelings Out

The other key to resolving trauma is finding ways to release trapped feelings related to it. The feelings we experience during a scary event often get locked up inside our bodies. We might want to scream when the bear is charging at us but don't because we need to stay hidden. We need to expel this traumatic energy from our systems. Sometimes we can release it by yelling and stomping our feet in a private, safe space, sometimes by crying in front of people who understand what happened to us, and sometimes by letting our bodies do the things they wanted to do but couldn't, like screaming while running as fast as we can into a safe place and then locking the door behind us.

Re-Parenting Our Younger Selves

One of my favorite "homework assignments" that I give to my clients with this type of trauma is to go find three pictures of themselves between infancy and five years old. I ask them to paste those pictures onto their bathroom mirrors and to have daily caring and nurturing conversations with their younger selves. It's healing to offer a younger you the comfort and affection that your caregivers weren't able to offer. No child is undeserving of love and attention. And when we start to recognize that and build a new perspective or story about our younger selves, the anxiety and depression related to our early neglect start to lift and be replaced by a secure sense of belonging.

This practice can change the narrative from "I was such an awkward and weird kid" to something like "I was so sweet and wanted so much to be loved, but since no one could help me feel that, I figured out how to entertain myself alone, surrounded by obscure action figures."

Once we can see ourselves as worthy kids who experienced neglect instead of weird kids who deserved isolation, the trauma moves from our bodies to our past. In trauma recovery the real flick of the wrist is in seeing ourselves with new eyes and honoring that we developed in a particular context that did not help us thrive.

Helping Ourselves Feel Safe

There's a big difference between being safe (no active threat to life, limb, or belonging) and actually *feeling* safe. When we feel traumatized or we're in the middle of a traumatic experience, our bodies are doing exactly what they need to by alerting us to the danger. They're sending "oh sh*t" signals all over our nervous systems to try to keep us safe.

However, when the traumatic event has ended but the trauma response in our bodies is still there, we need help learning how to feel safe. In practical terms, we need to take actions that encourage our brains and bodies to enter a calm or relaxed state.

WHEN IT ISN'T THAT SIMPLE

The bear-meets-grocery-store experience would be considered a single-incident trauma, which is sometimes even referred to as "simple" trauma because the thing that felt scary was overt and happened once. Single-incident trauma tends to heal faster and with more simplicity than more complex trauma. Complex trauma is a set of traumatic relationship dynamics or experiences that happen on repeat and over a prolonged period, especially during our childhood development. It's often also covert or confusing, making it harder to recognize, understand, and verbalize, making the narrative part of healing the trauma far more complicated to nail down.

For example, not knowing whether you're loved, wanted, or cherished by your family as you grow up would be considered complex trauma. Not feeling loved or wanted by a child's caregivers threatens their sense of belonging. Their nervous system is constantly in a heightened state, and they experience an anxious dread whenever they feel ignored, misunderstood, dismissed, etc. If a child feels unwanted or unloved, they likely experience the physical sensations associated with chronic anxiety and depression. These responses are not a choice. Children don't get to decide whether they feel emotionally safe or how they cope with it.

Complex trauma is a pile-up of moments of disconnection, neglect, or abuse that accumulate in a child's body and mind over time.

As complex trauma produces ongoing responses in a child's body, a trauma narrative starts to surround this reality. Since children do not have enough life experience to recognize that feeling unwanted is a neglect problem, their most likely conclusion is that they are unlikable or unworthy of love and affection.

The trauma variables in this situation would look something like:

- The traumatic experience: having parents who don't express delight, warmth, affection, or desire for connection
- The traumatic response: anxiety or depression
- The traumatic narrative: "Something is wrong with me."

If you relate to this section, the first thing I want to say to you is, "I'm so heartbroken that you went through that as a child. It was a truly harrowing and devastating trauma, even if you can't find a picture of it when you look up 'trauma' on Google. You didn't deserve to feel like that, I promise."

The second thing I want to say is that while we cannot go back and make our parents more affectionate or expressive of their love, or go back and remove the anxiety or depression we felt going through an emotionally neglectful dynamic, we can work to rewrite the story we tell ourselves about what happened to us. We can decide to change the story from "something was wrong with me" to "some things were wrong or inadequate with the environment I grew up in."

Sensory Shifting Interventions

We can use our senses to help our bodies "sense" the safety of the room we're in with:

- Smells—such as oils, candles, or nature scents (I love cracking open a pine needle and taking in the aroma.)
- Touch—such as soft blankets, fidget toys, or even play dough-can help give us tactile input that helps us to feel calmer
- Sounds—music, nature noises, or the absence of sound can give our minds "background" feelings that helps us to relax
- Visuals—dimming or increasing lights or looking at beautiful pictures can give us something reassuring or beautiful to focus on that help our minds to redirect our feelings of fear or panic
- Taste—eating something can help us get calmer by reminding us we have the safety of food to nourish our bodies

Relationship-Based Interventions

We can ask others to help us feel safe by:

- Asking for assurance that they're feeling safe in the same room as us
- Asking to be held or hugged while we work to absorb the calmness and care of another person
- Asking for space to think or reflect if we're feeling overwhelmed or overstimulated
- Asking for someone to distract us long enough to get our bodies into a less tense or scared state

Take It Slow

Healing from trauma is rarely a hundred-meter dash. Our bodies usually need time to process the feelings, images, and beliefs that our trauma has tangled around us and our relationships. If you recognize this is something you need to deal with, please give yourself permission to go at whatever pace your heart and body need you to. Trauma happens to us in the blink of an eye without our consent, so it's fundamentally healing to give ourselves a thoughtful and paced process to heal through it.

Take It to Therapy

I obviously have a bias here—I'm a shrink for heaven's sake! *But* I've also been a client and have had my fair share of complex trauma that I had to excavate and heal to feel safe and secure in the present.

I think it's a very wise move to take our big and complicated trauma stories to therapy instead of trying to white knuckle through them on our own. When we have a good therapist, we can utilize their expertise and care to help us traverse terrain that is often emotionally swampy and hard to walk through alone.

I want to acknowledge that being able to access and afford therapy, both in financial terms and also in terms of time, is a privilege that not everyone has. The more time and money we have access to, the easier it is to connect with a therapist who's a good fit for us.

But I hope that doesn't dissuade you from trying to find the therapy you need. Check page 267 for tips on finding accessible, affordable, and culturally competent therapy that works for you.

Modeling Hope

It takes true courage to acknowledge that we're feeling traumatized, especially if that feeling has lingered in our bodies for years. But healing our stuck trauma is one of the most important things we can do for our children and their relationships with us.

When we put in the work to deal with feeling traumatized, it models that healing and hope are also possible for our children. Even though we hope they won't, our children will likely face some form of trauma in their lives, and what a tremendous advantage they'll have if they've already seen us walk a path of recovery from our own trauma.

Compassionate Self-Talk Scripts

- *"I am not what has happened to me. I am all the ways I survived it and now all the ways I'm healing from it."*
- *"It makes sense that I feel scared or unsafe in situations that remind me of past trauma. I can ask for support from people who love me to help me process those feelings, even when they're surfacing in situations where I am technically safe."*
- *"I deserve relationships in which people respect my boundaries, are gentle with my feelings, and are able to understand me."*

Trusty Tidbit

CREATIVE PLAY FOR FEELING SAFE(R)

The opposite of feeling traumatized is not feeling safe—it's feeling playful or creative.

Think of the spectrum like this:

I AM VERY SCARED
I AM LESS SCARED
I AM SAFE
I AM EMPOWERED
I AM PLAYING OR CREATING

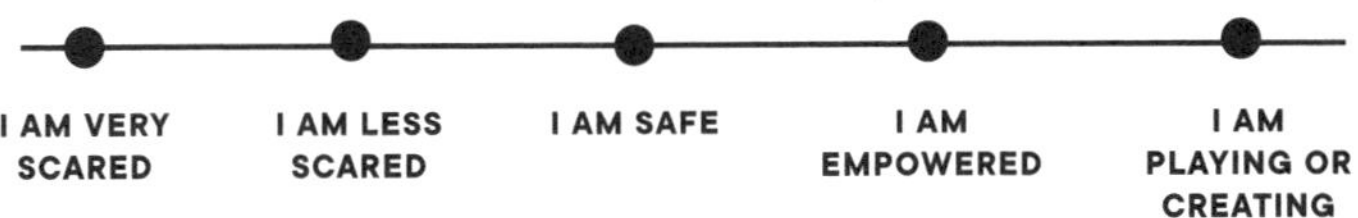

Healing from trauma is more than facing the hard stories we have lived; it's also claiming our capacity for creativity. When the past tries to take over the present, paint, sing, dance, write, play dress up, cook, and feel how alive you are in that moment.

Further Reading

Body-First Healing: Get Unstuck and Recover from Trauma with Somatic Healing by Brittany Piper

Emotional Inheritance by Dr. Galit Atlas

Homecoming: Healing Trauma to Reclaim Your Authentic Self by Thema Bryant

No Bad Parts: Healing Trauma and Restoring Wholeness with the Internal Family Systems Model by Richard Schwartz

Trauma and Recovery: The Aftermath of Violence—from Domestic Abuse to Political Terror by Judith Lewis Herman, MD

Waking the Tiger: Healing Trauma by Peter A. Levine

Why Am I Like This?: How to Break Cycles, Heal from Trauma, and Restore Your Faith by Kobe Campbell

II: The Habits

The most impactful lessons we teach our children are the ones they learn from watching us live. Our habits and actions are the most accurate picture of our emotional capacity, and the ways we consistently act will ultimately lead our children to conclude that we are, or are not, a secure place for them.

Which is why our negative habits need our attention. Emotional maturity is partly learning how to feel and partly learning how to respond maturely to our feelings. Which means ditching problematic coping habits.

Having bad habits does not make us bad people or bad parents, but it can put our relationships with our children under serious strain. For most of us, the path toward secure relationships with our children involves working to discard insecure habits that prevent us from developing more emotionally mature patterns.

I chose to focus on the particular habits in this next section because they're the most common and damaging habits that I've seen wreak havoc on the five gifts in my life, the lives of my therapy clients, and the lives of my friends and family.

We develop these habits in response to the emotions, relationships, and traumatic experiences that we didn't know how to navigate. At certain points in our journeys, these habits were the best coping skills we had access to. They were a strategic way to survive a landscape of disconnection, trauma, emotional chaos, or loss. We used these habits to cope either because we *didn't have the power to change a dynamic or situation* or because *we didn't yet have the insight or supportive resources that we needed to feel empowered to create change*. But now it's time to outgrow them.

These habits come in three different forms:

Mental habits are the habits we utilize to think and develop meaning about important things. Although our mental habits occur within our minds, they have a huge external impact on how we behave and relate. Our mental habits can develop as a result of things we were taught growing up or from our own conclusions about ourselves and the world as a result of our experiences. Our kids study our mental states for cues that we're available to them, that we see them accurately, and that we're regulated enough to handle what they need from us. When we're stuck in negative mental habits, our children tend to steer clear of our minds instead of finding refuge in them.

Coping habits are the behavioral habits we utilize when we're feeling emotionally overwhelmed. These are the things we do to get through emotional pain. Coping habits can be positive or negative, and some are a bit of both. The ones I've chosen to write about here are generally net negative, which is why they need our attention.

When we cope by either shutting down or trying to grasp for control, we demonstrate to our children that we haven't yet learned how to tolerate our emotional responses. Our kids can't seek us out for understanding, delight, and belonging if they anticipate that we'll either overreact or underreact to their emotions.

Relational habits are the things we do in response to others, especially in our closest relationships. Our relational habits obviously have a massive impact on our children. How emotionally open or closed we are, how calm or reactive, and how confident or insecure we are can affect how many of the five gifts our children can receive from us.

Some of these habits have only one element from the list above, others will hit all three. The more integrated a habit is into our mindsets, behaviors, and relational patterns, the more damaging it is to the security of our relationships with our children. And unfortunately the harder it is to change. As you read each section, ask yourself whether that habit plays a role in how you think, act, and relate. If you find one that's hitting all three, I advise you to give that particular habit some serious attention before moving on to the other chapters.

If shame starts to get in the way (it almost always does), head back to the section on shame to care for that emotional state so you can regulate your heart and mind and get back to work breaking whatever habit you're tackling.

When Habits Are Traditions

Some of our habits are family traditions. They may have formed in recent generations or developed over centuries. This makes our process of change far more complicated, because we're not only changing a habit, we are breaking with tradition. If this is true for you, I encourage you to build a support team to help you through your habit-breaking journey.

As social animals we need to know that we belong, and when we break with family traditions, even the unspoken ones such as drinking profusely, talking negatively about ourselves, or striving for perfection, it can shift our position of acceptance and belonging within our families of origin. Belonging with other cycle-breakers who share our determination to heal generational trauma can help to curb the panic we feel when we move away from accepted family traditions that do not serve our children or our relationships with them.

On the other hand, some of our habits are our personal rebellions against family traditions. These are the things we do to resist whatever family inheritance we found unhelpful or intolerable growing up. I know quite a few people who grew up as members of strict religions and developed serious drug and alcohol habits as rebellious responses. I also know people who grew up in homes with serious drug and alcohol habits who developed rigid control mindsets as a corrective response.

No matter if our habits are a continuation of family traditions or a rebellion against them, the important thing is that we're honest with ourselves about the presence of these habits in our lives and the negative impact they're having.

Ask Yourself

With any habits in our lives, it's important to ask ourselves:

Does this habit help or hinder my ability to . . .

1. Show my children I can handle their emotions?
2. Show my children I understand their perspectives?
3. Show my children that I want to be close to them?
4. Show up for my children when they need me?
5. Show my children that I accept them for their full, authentic selves?

Regardless of their origins we want to uproot any relational habits that cultivate disconnection, misunderstanding, and overbearing dynamics.

Habits are hard to break, but I hope we all choose to break our bad habits instead of breaking our children's hearts. When I think about it in those terms, it really helps me keep my priorities straight.

Imagine the habits you wished your parents had broken. Imagine them breaking them even now. It would be a gift to you, right? It's never too late, and it's always a huge relief both to the parent and the child.

Let's start breaking some wonky habits!!

How to Deal with a Control Habit

"You are worthy of love, belonging, dignity, and respect. You don't have to earn any of it. Neither do your children."

—JOHN FOGEL, *Punishment-Free Parenting*

A control habit comes from the incredibly burdensome belief that if we don't make things happen in a very particular way, some unknown terrible thing might happen. Plus the sister belief that it's good for our children to learn to submit to authority. This habit fixates our relational patterns onto dominance and control instead of connection and collaboration ("I'm the boss!! You will do what I say! If you don't, something bad might happen to you or to me!").

When we get stuck in this habit, it's *usually* not because we're power-yielding overlords who enjoy dominating our children. (Though sadly parents with that level of psychological disturbance do exist.) Most of us struggle with this habit because we're afraid our children will be "out of control" if we don't try to control them.

So many of us were brought up in homes or communities that were focused on control through fear ("Who is right?" "Who is winning?" "Who has the approval of the people in charge?"

"What bad things will happen if we don't do this right or perfectly?"). These experiences shaped our understanding of what's important, leading us to fear loss of control and to misunderstand our roles in helping our children develop resilience.

When we're stuck in a control habit, the question "Is my child doing what I think they should?" feels more important than the question "Is my child getting what they need in their relationship with me?"

This looks like:

- Fixating on compliance and obedience without considering our children's needs, developmental stage, or capacity
- Interpreting our children's questioning or pushback as defiance or disrespect
- Involving ourselves in all decisions and constantly checking on progress
- Moving quickly to anger when our children do things we don't like
- Guilt-tripping (see page 202) to gain compliance with our wishes
- Requiring that our children apologize to us first to show submission to our authority
- Utilizing tools of control, such as shame and punishment, when we want to change our children's behavior

How Does a Control Habit Affect Our Children?

A control habit can get in the way of gifts #1, 2, and 5 of a secure parent (page x). If we habitually seek control in our relationships with our children, we can't respond effectively to their emotions (gift #1), listen respectfully to their perspectives (gift #2), or show them we want them to be their full, authentic selves (gift #5).

My mom's father, Jim Stone, or "Grandpa Honey" as we called him growing up, was not the type of grandpa that his nickname implied. We called him Grandpa Honey because both my grandfathers were named Jim, so we referred to each of them by the names of their dogs to avoid confusion. Unfortunately, because of a rampant control habit, time with Grandpa Honey felt anything but sweet.

My childhood memories of him mostly involve feeling scared, teased, or sore. Scared because he would rage at us or humiliate us if we didn't fall in line with whatever he thought was right. Teased because the only way he allowed himself to "play" with us was to make fun of what we were wearing or saying, or how we chose to style our hair. And sore? Because he had a disfigured and very stiff middle finger that he had caught in a combine when he was a child, and he used it to knock us over our heads whenever he came to visit. The only time I ever saw Grandpa Honey laugh was when one of us cried or grimaced in response to this repeated finger thumping.

I have no memories of Grandpa Honey hugging me, listening to me, encouraging me, or saying anything affectionate in my direction. All my memories involve him exerting his authority over me and trying to get me to act, think, or dress however he thought was best for me (and doing the same to everyone else in the room).

I have a memory of my three-year-old brother putting his elbows on the table and my grandfather erupting in rage at him, pounding his hands on the dinner table so aggressively that the silverware jumped in fear of him. He was so concerned with controlling our behavior that he was often out of control himself.

I have inklings as to why Grandpa Honey was so controlling. He was raised by a father who had a very serious drinking problem and a mother who had survived a cult situation and estranged herself from her entire family, causing her to be very cold and controlling herself. My grandfather's only relational refuge had been with his older brother, who had passed away unexpectedly when he was still a kid. It makes sense that he struggled to be vulnerable and connected and instead got caught up in a control habit.

Tragically for him and for us, he was so focused on controlling our behavior that he was never able to be warm, connected, or compassionate, which meant we never developed a meaningful relationship with him. His impulse toward control suffocated any opportunity for anyone to be authentically safe and connected in his presence.

A focus on controlling our children has three very serious side effects on their lives:

1. It alienates them from our support. When we're focused on controlling our children, they learn to hide their struggles from us. Instead of utilizing our guidance and emotional comfort, they try to please us and bury their more complicated needs inside themselves or in relationships outside of our homes.
2. It teaches them to be compliant when they have less power than someone else. Unfortunately this is a very dangerous habit for them. They'll come across many people and institutions in their lifetimes that have harmful agendas and intentions toward them. If we've bathed them in an authoritarian dynamic with us, they won't have the skills for negotiation and self-advocacy that they'll need later on to stand up to injustice or to walk away from abuse.

3. It leads to them feeling traumatized in their relationships with us. Our relationships with our parents are where we seek support, safety, and belonging. If a parent has an authoritarian habit, it makes it hard for them to meet any of those needs. Instead we fear being rejected or in trouble, which can be not only painful, but can inflict a sense of threat on our nervous systems.

Most of us who struggle with control habits aren't as entrenched in them as Grandpa Honey was. But even if we are, we can choose to change the habit and learn how to step out of control-based relational patterns and build connection-based relationship dynamics with our children.

Let's Grow!

A control habit is driven by deep anxiety and/or authoritarian beliefs about our roles as parents, so it's broken by a combination of dealing with our anxiety (see page 21 on how to deal with anxiety) and switching our mindsets to being connection-focused. Here's how to make the switch:

Keep Your Eyes On the Prize

Our children are life's most generous gift, and the experience of having a front row seat as their parents is truly sacred. We must remind ourselves regularly that our goal is to be a supportive character in our children's journey, not the narrator or even the writer. Because if we try to write their story, we'll be in the way of their own writing process, and they'll eventually have to push us aside to do whatever they need to do to live the lives they are born to live.

Repeat after me: *"No amount of control or structure is worth losing the opportunity to be authentically close with my child."*

Learn to Tolerate Vulnerability and Uncertainty

One of the most important skills we can develop to strengthen our relationships with our children is the ability to tolerate our feelings of vulnerability and uncertainty. These feelings are not just part of childhood, they're a normal part of parenthood too. When we learn how to feel them without immediately grasping for control, we become far more trustworthy to our children.

Repeat after me: *"I can work to gain control over my child, ultimately losing connection and influence with them, or I can learn to tolerate the vulnerability and uncertainty that often arise in parenting and learn to hold both my mind and my child's mind in my heart at the same time."*

Learn to Be Both Solid and Flexible

We don't have to be in charge of everything to be in charge of some things. And part of our jobs as parents is to slowly relinquish control and responsibility over to our children as they gain the skills needed to take over tasks. (I'm no longer a part of wiping any of my children's butts, and I feel so good about this!!!)

When we're stuck controlling things that our children can handle themselves, we hinder them from learning important lessons. They need to take things on to discover what they're capable of and sometimes to face natural consequences that help them learn important lessons.

Sharing power and voice with our children doesn't mean we flip the script and put them in charge of everything. It means we intentionally recognize when they're ready to handle increased autonomy, responsibility, or influence in their lives, and entrust them with opportunities to learn.

Trusty Tidbit

I DON'T KNOW EVERYTHING

Parents who can acknowledge that they don't know everything are more effective in maintaining a position as an advisor and consultant with their children as they age.

"I don't know" is a perfectly secure thing to say to our children. By modeling that we're not all-knowing, we're building trust with our children about the things we do know.

It can also be followed up with, "Let's see how we can learn that together." Learning alongside each other is an incredibly rich way to bond.

Repeat after me:

"I can cultivate cooperation by showing my children that I care about what they feel and letting them have a voice and choice in areas of our shared life that they're ready to handle."

"I can trust myself and my children to (mostly) make good decisions, and when mistakes are made, I want to foster the belief in my children that I'm approachable and supportive."

Further Reading

Break the Cycle: A Guide to Healing Intergenerational Trauma by Dr. Mariel Buqué

Parenting Beyond Power: How to Use Connection and Collaboration to Transform Your Family—and the World by Jen Lumanlan, MS, MEd

Punishment-Free Parenting: The Brain-Based Way to Raise Kids Without Raising Your Voice by Jon Fogel

How to Deal with a Bias Habit

"Distance breeds suspicion. But proximity breeds empathy."

—TYLER MERRITT, *I Take My Coffee Black*

I feel nervous writing this section of the book. We're living through incredibly polarized times. Hate is on the rise, and we're being conditioned by political strategists, marketing teams, and publicists to see each other in extreme caricatures.

We are losing our grip on peaceful civil discourse and on shared commitment to show respect for each other's humanity, especially when we disagree or come from different vantage points.

But since I believe it's our job as parents to be people our children can look up to, I'm going to remain hopeful that we can figure out how to deal with our biases enough to make this situation better for our children.

In the wise words of James Baldwin, "Children have never been very good at listening to their elders, but they have never failed to imitate them." Our children are closely watching how we talk about and relate to people who are different from us. We can't expect our children to be kind, patient, and curious with others if we're not doing so ourselves.

What Exactly Is a Bias Habit?

The University of Chicago defines "bias" as "a natural inclination for or against an idea, object, group, or individual."

I grew up believing that only bad guys had biases because I thought bias and bigotry were the same thing. If you'd asked me about my biases in my younger adult years, I would have been offended and exclaimed, *"No, Ma'am! I'm not biased against anyone! I'm one of the good guys who believe all people are created equal!"* I thought that admitting bias would mean I was someone who lived with active hate in my heart, like the members of the Ku Klux Klan.

But what I have learned over the years studying human relationships is that the more work we do to acknowledge and examine our biases, the less likely we are to develop entrenched prejudices or act out cruelty toward others.

We all seek proximity to people who look, feel, and think like us for safety and belonging. We're primed to see ourselves as part of a group and to value the interests of that group as a part of our survival strategy. That is only a problem because it also means that we naturally feel skeptical of people who look, feel, and think differently from us as a way to protect ourselves from both threat and rejection.

Our ancestors' instinct to see people similar to them as good and foreigners as bad served their survival when they were foraging for food or faced with nefarious strangers with intent to invade.

But eventually our ancestors figured out that we could pool our resources and knowledge together and innovate more efficient strategies to support larger communities. Which is why I am writing on a laptop that is made of diverse materials harvested from locations all over the globe. At this point in human history we are a global community, which means that our biases for or against smaller subsections of people no longer serve us. Whether we like it or not, we are all in this together from this point forward.

Unfortunately, when we feel afraid, there is still an ancient instinct in our bones to blame outsiders for our problems. And when we project blame outside of ourselves and people like us and onto those we don't know well, we can stoke the fires of our natural biases and grow them into bigotry.

Bigotry is when we not only ignore our biases or deny that we have them, but we *invest in our biases and feed them* until they grow into strong feelings of fear, resentment, and hatred toward others. A bigot is defined by the Britannica Dictionary as, "a person who hates or refuses to accept the members of a particular group (such as a racial or religious group)."

I think of bias as a small infection of misinformation and misunderstanding about an unfamiliar group of people, while bigotry is a septic infection. If we deal with our biases before they turn to bigotry, there will be much less damage to ourselves and to anyone who is different from us.

Acknowledging Our Biases Is the First Step Toward Preventing Harm

Well-respected research has proven that we *all* have biases and that our biases are often unconsciously driving our choices. This means it's common for us to be unintentionally unfair to our fellow human beings.

I find this simultaneously reassuring *and* disturbing. Reassuring because it means our biases don't make us bad people. Disturbing because it means everyone has biases inside them, and that means there are billions of opportunities for biases to turn into accidental or intentional exclusion or bigotry.

While we can't control what other people do with their biases, we can certainly take responsibility for what we do with ours.

Specifically, we can choose to dismantle our biases and take a journey toward greater curiosity, humility, and openness to people who are different from ourselves. Our biases only become problems when we choose not to examine them or when we feed them with fearful or hateful misinformation and let them grow into bigotry.

How Our Unexamined Biases Affect Our Children

How our biases affect our children depends on whether we choose to:

Ignore our biases and deny that we have them: This leads our children to be unsure about how we feel about people who are different from us. The "ignore" approach doesn't eliminate our biases, it just keeps them unspoken. Instead of learning about our biases in an overt way, our children will learn about them through our unconscious choices. Our biases are evident through who we spend time with, who we avoid, what books, films, social media, and art we consume, and how we talk (or don't talk) about people who are different from us. Our indifference toward our biases validates them in our children's eyes, even if we never talk about them explicitly.

Attempt to justify our biases: And if we cultivate the reasons we don't like particular groups of people (turning bias into prejudice), our children may learn to do the same, perpetuating the bias further into the world. This is how hate gets its wings and is passed down from one generation to the next.

Or if our children don't inherit our hate, they'll likely start to distance themselves from us. They'll fear telling us the truth about any significant connections they develop with people we feel biased against. And they'll be even more scared to let us know if they see themselves as part of a group they have experienced our biases against.

If we take that prejudice to the next level and become active in political or social groups that identify themselves by *who they're against*, then we're in much bigger trouble. Not only will our children struggle to be honest with us about their potential identities and connections, but they'll also lose respect for us and start to create distance from us, because hate is the opposite of emotional maturity and security.

When we allow bias to take center stage in our interactions with others, we're limiting how we view both others and ourselves. And when it comes to our children, we're teaching them they must choose between who they know themselves to be (or who they know others to be) and our love and approval. This is a terrible and unfixable conundrum.

Some of our children will choose themselves and sever their connections with us. Others will choose us and will lose an important part of themselves in the process. And most tragically, some will decide they can't bear the cost of living with the tension of that choice and will choose to leave the world altogether. (According to the Trevor Project, 39 percent of LGBTQ youths have seriously considered suicide in the last year, including 46 percent of transgender and nonbinary youths.)

Most of us will never don a white pointy hat and consciously participate in the murder and dehumanization of other human beings. But that doesn't mean our unexamined or accepted biases aren't detrimental to the lives of our children. Even without us realizing it.

Many of us will have children who identify as people with beliefs and identities that we have biases against. We'll also likely have children who love people who belong to groups that we hold biases toward. Not to mention the fact that our children have their own minds, and as they grow they will develop their own unique sets of beliefs and values. If we want to stay authentically close with our children throughout their lives, we need to be willing to notice and challenge whatever biases we've developed.

Keep in mind that our biases play out differently in each of our homes, depending on our cultural backgrounds, life experiences, religious upbringings, and the systems we're part of.

Examples of How Our Biases Can Show Up in Our Parenting

- Assuming a child's future intelligence, interests, or career is based on their gender (girls aren't good at math, boys can't be nurturing or stay-at-home parents, etc.)
- Discouraging certain friendships or activities because of discomfort with stereotypes about class, religion, or culture
- Mocking people's accents on television or in real life
- Praising people's thinness or weight loss on television or in real life (also see How to Deal with Feeling Body Disgust, page 39)
- Idealizing traits, behavior, and styles that are linked with "whiteness" or social class—lighter skin, straighter hair, "proper" speech—as more attractive or successful
- Interrupting or dismissing a child's emotion because of their gender (for example, boys are weak when they cry or girls are dramatic if they're angry)
- Insisting our children wear certain colors or clothing based on gender, despite their protests

- Avoiding difficult conversations about race, gender, or injustice because "it makes kids feel uncomfortable," especially with children who don't hold vulnerable positions around those topics
- Talking about other people's religious beliefs as weird or inferior
- Mocking other people's languages, traditions, foods, or other parts of their culture
- Justifying harm to others (war, famine, etc.) based on the cultural identity of that group
- Talking about certain groups of people as "those" people—immigrants, LGBTQ+ folks, people with disabilities—instead of using the groups' preferred ways of being identified
- Assuming our children's sexuality when talking about potential crushes and dating
- Making judgments about someone's parenting, intelligence, or worthiness based on what they wear, how they speak, or where they live
- Pressuring children to "fit in" or capitulate to peer pressure, especially when fitting in means erasing parts of their identity
- Talking about our racial or cultural identity as superior to other groups

Trusty Tidbit

LEARNING TO UNLEARN

When we recognize we're wrong about someone based on a stereotype, we can choose to shift how we view that person and their group and to change the way we approach anyone whom we know very little about. My stepfather told me about a time when he was faced with his bias as a young man and asked if he could share it with us here:

> As a Chinese American biracial person, I was no stranger to knowing that many people were prejudiced in the world when I was growing up. My Chinese mother often talked disparagingly about other Asian races that she saw as lesser than us, and I was determined never to be prejudiced in the same way. But one day in my early adulthood, I was visiting some family friends, and they wanted to introduce me to a new priest in their church. On the way to meet him, my friends told me that he was Latino. I had visions in my head about what that would mean about this priest. All my visions were based on the Latino day workers whom I had seen at the local convenience store in Virginia. The biases in my mind led me to imagine he would be shorter and less educated than me. When he walked into the room, he not only physically towered over me, but I learned that he also had a PhD from the Sorbonne and could mop the floor with me in terms of both intellect and education. That day I realized how incredibly inaccurate my beliefs could be about a people group I had had very little interpersonal interactions with. And I promised myself from then onward that I would always rethink my initial assumptions about people, especially about people with whom I had very little previous exposure."

Let's Grow!

The first step toward overcoming our biases is to acknowledge they exist.

We can ask ourselves:

- What groups of people do I have little or no personal exposure to?
- What groups of people am I uncomfortable seeing or interacting with?
- What groups of people have I been taught to mistrust, fear, or look down upon?
- When I choose to watch TV or read a book, what groups of people are never in my lineup of stories?

Busting Our Biases with Proximity and Empathy

The opposite of bias against someone is the empathy that comes from understanding more about them. Allowing ourselves to feel empathetic toward someone means allowing ourselves to connect to their humanity. Instead of looking down at someone or looking away from their reality, we connect to what they're experiencing in the world. But we can't have empathy for people we never get to know, either through their stories or through real-life encounters with them.

The first step toward busting up our biases is to deepen our understanding and proximity to people we feel uncomfortable with. We can do that by:

- Reading books written by people we know we're biased against
- Watching films and movies written by and portraying the stories of people we feel biased against

- Taking time to listen to podcasts and read articles written by people in the group we're biased against, who are explaining the perspectives or life conditions of that group
- Visiting restaurants and cultural centers of a people group to learn about all of the ways they live and to notice their similarities to us, as well as things we can learn from them
- Following the social media accounts of people from groups we do not belong to

The more we expose ourselves to people we don't understand, the more we can gain the understanding we need to develop a respectful approach to them.

INTERNALIZED SELF-BIAS

When we grow up in cultures or families that hold negative views about us, we can internalize those views and develop a bias against ourselves. This bias usually surfaces as negative feelings about how our bodies look, function, or feel. (see page 39 about how -isms can create body disgust). It's equally important to evaluate our self-biases as it is our biases against others.

Dig into Education About Bias Breaking

The more we recognize that we have biases and work to dismantle them through curiosity and learning, the more our children will see us as compassionate and wise supports in their lives. And the more likely they'll be honest with us about who they are, who they love, and how they see the world.

The Further Reading in this section will help you continue to grow as someone who takes responsibility over their biases and, therefore, as someone your children can trust to be accepting, curious, and open to new people and ideas.

Compassionate Self-Talk Scripts

- *"Just because I hold a bias against a group of people doesn't mean my opinions are true. It also doesn't mean that I am a terrible person myself. It means that I have something to learn."*
- *"Feeling scared to talk about biases and differences is normal. It's vulnerable to walk into complicated topics, especially with people I care about."*
- *"My children are not supposed to be everything I want; they're supposed to be everything they want. I can learn how to love them for who they are, even if I don't understand it at first."*

Further Reading

Free to Be: Understand Kids and Gender Identity by Jack Turban, MD
How to Raise an Antiracist by Ibram X. Kendi
I Take My Coffee Black by Tyler Merritt
Parenting with Pride by Heather Hester
Raising Critical Thinkers: A Parent's Guide to Growing Wise Kids in the Digital Age by Julie Bogart
The Person You Mean to Be: How Good People Fight Bias by Dolly Chugh

How to Deal with a Blaming Habit

"The way we talk to our children becomes their inner voice."
—PEGGY O'MARA

If something goes wrong, does it always feel like it has to be someone's fault? Well that's what happens in a family where a parent has a blaming habit. If something spills or is missing, or there's a conflict between siblings, the habitual response is for the parent to launch an investigation to find out who's to blame. Who started it? Who messed up? Someone needs to fess up and then pay up.

A blaming habit is closely related to a control habit (page 160). It stems from the notion that the authority in the room needs to use their power to control those on the lower rungs of the ladder.

It took me a while to shake this habit and to learn to see messes and conflicts through a "needs" lens rather than a "fault" lens. My parents unintentionally modeled a blame habit for me when I was growing up, eventually getting divorced when I was sixteen. Before their marriage ended, I watched as they regularly engaged in battles over who was at fault. These arguments became emotionally tense very quickly, and the tension could remain for long periods.

I didn't realize until I was raising my kids that I used a people-pleasing habit (page 224) to avoid the painful experience of feeling blamed. I felt defensive (page 51) when people gave me any form of negative feedback about how I had impacted them. And internally I found ways to ensure the blame landed on other people and not on me.

But when my children were toddlers and the unavoidable sibling spats began, I realized this habit wasn't going to serve them or me, and I had to figure out how to do things differently.

How Does a Blaming Habit Affect Our Children?

A blaming habit is damaging to our children's sense of security in their relationships with us. It mucks up the secure parent gift #2, trusting that we understand their perspective, and gift #4, feeling that we can show up for them when they need us. If our children sense that mistakes and emotional dysregulation will be met with blame, they have to contend with either shame ("What's wrong with me?") or defensiveness ("It wasn't my fault!!!"). And neither of those things helps children develop true responsibility.

Blame teaches children how to avoid being blamed and how to blame themselves and others. And when they grow up, it makes it harder for them to take responsibility without feeling panic or shame. This makes it more common for them to blame other people (including us) for their problems instead of seeking solutions for themselves.

Personal responsibility is born out of feeling empowered and guided, not blamed.

Let's Grow!

Instead of blaming ourselves or our children when things go awry, we can pivot into a *respond* and *account* approach.

It's helpful to break down the roots of the words "responsibility" and "accountability" to get to the heart of what they each mean. These words share the same suffix "ability," which refers to *the ability to do something*. The prefix of "responsibility" is "response" or "respond," meaning "to answer." And the prefix of "accountability" is to "count" or "report." (And an "accountant" is someone whose job is to reconcile data into coherent conclusions.)

If we want to help our children learn accountability and responsibility, we need to focus on helping them learn *how to be responsive* and then *how to reconcile their behavior with its impact*.

These are not simple skills. They're skills that develop over time and require a ton of support. Here's how we help them do it:

Model, Model, Model

We are the models. How we act in response to other people's pain or in response to conflict are the templates our children will learn most potently. For them to learn what responsibility and accountability look like, they need to witness us do two primary things:

1. Be receptive and responsive when people tell us we impacted them negatively. Let's say we accidentally cut someone off while driving in traffic, and they honk at us to prevent us from causing a collision. If we're modeling responsibility, we say out loud (even if the other driver can't hear us), "Aaaaaack, I'm so sorry! Thank you for honking and keeping us from getting into a fender bender!"
2. Actively take an account of how our actions impacted someone else. Once we're past the adrenaline rush, we need to narrate

to our children what happened and how we impacted the situation. "Oof, I really didn't do a good job of checking my blind spot, and I almost knocked knuckles with that other driver. Thank goodness they honked, and I was able to swerve away and avoid an accident."

When we showcase ourselves responding to others whom we've negatively impacted, and then describe the situation in a way that's neither self-depreciating nor defensive, it demonstrates to our children that it's possible to be responsible and accountable. And when our children get to witness how incredibly effective it is to do these things with them or other people in our lives, it makes responsibility and accountability desirable. A trend the human race is in desperate need of.

Obviously we can't do this all the time. Sometimes the other driver goes ballistic and flashes us the bird while flailing out their window, making it harder to stay present with our mistake because we're now processing their out-of-control response to it. But even if we're not perfect at this, we can be consistent. And it can be in simple situations, such as accidentally stepping on our dog's tail, making them yelp. We can respond with, "Oh no, Brutus, so sorry, pal!" and then model for our kids that we can acknowledge we hurt Brutus because we weren't looking where we were walking, and we feel awful that he got hurt.

Reach Before You Teach

When our children do things that cause harm to others (or to our carpets), they need us to help them understand what happened. Which means we have to pause and reflect on the situation first. Sometimes when my kids have done something I don't like, I physically leave the room for a few minutes before I respond. It helps me to put a barrier between me and the impulse to resort to blame mode.

I ask myself, "Why did my child do this, and how can I help them learn from it?" I always answer the first question in a way that honors my child's dignity. Our children are doing the best they can in the moment, and being harsh toward them doesn't help them learn to do better; it simply teaches them to hide their mistakes more effectively.

Once I have an idea of why they did it (perhaps they're still learning to manage their anger, they had an impulse they didn't know how to control, or they truly didn't think there was a problem with what they did and they need education), I return to the room and respond to their underlying motivation.

I'm responding first because that's what I want them to learn—to consider the motivations and feelings of others. By doing that with them, they get to explore themselves in a way that helps them eventually develop greater curiosity for their inner worlds and the inner worlds of others.

Let's say they angrily threw a hula hoop at their dad after he tried to teach them the very sophisticated "flick of the wrist" involved in throwing the hoop forward and getting it to roll backward. (Okay, you caught me, this literally happened in my house last night.) My husband maturely walked away after getting walloped in the noggin to keep from reacting strongly, and I went to my child and said, "Is learning how to hula hoop bringing feelings of frustration into your body?" She confirmed this was the case. I opened my arms to her and held her while she sobbed, "I'm stupid, I can't do this." I replied, "Those are some big, overwhelming shame feelings you're having. I get them too sometimes when I'm learning something new." We sat for a minute while she cried in my arms until her body relaxed, and I could sense that she had the responsiveness she needed from me to shift into accounting mode.

"I think Dad was trying to help you learn, and it probably really hurt his head and his heart when he got smacked by the hoop. Do you think that's true?" She was regulated enough to process the information without getting defensive and immediately went to find my husband and apologize.

Because we avoided blaming her ("Bad girl, look what you did to your poor father who was just trying to help you!!!"), she could process herself and move toward reconciliation with very little prompting or instruction.

Breaking a blame habit becomes much easier when we remember that blame is a way to harness control, not a way to help a child learn how to be responsive and accountable for their impact in the world.

Blame Changers

Use these simple script changes to reduce blame and increase curiosity, compassion, and understanding:

- "Who did this?" ⟶ "What happened here?"
- "You're in big trouble, mister!" ⟶ "I'm going to help you make this right."
- "Look what you did!!!" ⟶ "I see what happened, and I'm here to help you figure it out."
- "Who started it?" ⟶ "Let's figure out what's going on for both of you and what you each need."

Compassionate Self-Talk Scripts

- *"Everyone is doing the best they can, including me."*
- *"My job isn't to find a culprit, it's to be an understanding and supportive guide."*
- *"I don't have to find fault to identify the things my children need my help to learn."*

Trusty Tidbit

RIGHT SIZING OUR RESPONSIBILITY

Just as we can have distorted views on our body size or shape (called "body dysmorphia" in the fancy psychology vernacular), we can also have "responsibility dysmorphia."

Sometimes our sense of responsibility is too big, leading us to mistakenly believe we're responsible for things that are not in our control.

Sometimes our sense of responsibility is too small, and we mistakenly think that it has to be someone else's fault alone.

We need to "right-size" our responsibility so that we accurately notice the ways we've impacted a situation or person.

If you have a responsibility dysmorphia on either side of the spectrum, work on either shrinking or growing your sense of responsibility. Adjust it to the right size to stop you from getting caught in a blame drain.

Further Reading

Grit: The Power of Passion and Perseverance by Angela Duckworth

Radical Responsibility: How to Move Beyond Blame, Fearlessly Live Your Highest Purpose, and Become an Unstoppable Force for Good by Fleet Maull, PhD, foreword by Daniel Siegel, MD

The Four Agreements: A Practical Guide to Personal Freedom by Don Miguel Ruiz

How to Deal with a Toxic Comparison Habit

"Here's my hunch: nobody's secure, and nobody feels like she completely belongs. Those insecurities are just job hazards of being human. But some people dance anyway, and those people have more fun."

—GLENNON DOYLE, *Carry On, Warrior*

It is *so hard* not to compare ourselves and our children to other people. It's hard because it's natural to pay attention to the people we encounter and to notice details about them in comparison to ourselves. We're wired as social creatures to assess others for the purposes of learning, safety, and belonging.

I like to imagine one of my ancestors in a cave somewhere in Ireland noticing a friend using a sharp rock to cut meat for her children and thinking, "This is brilliant, I've got to have one of my own!!" She asks her friend where she got the rock, goes out and finds one for her family, and increases her ability to utilize valuable protein before it rots. Social comparison helped our cave-dwelling predecessors acquire adaptive tools and practices that kept them alive. I like to think of this as an *advantageous* comparison.

But unfortunately for all of us, not all comparison is advantageous. We can get caught up in a toxic cycle of comparison that keeps us loaded with insecurity and anxiety instead of improving our survival skills.

Let's Grow!

Comparison can leave us feeling that we need more, more, more in order to feel that we have enough. This is a problem for us and our children because it means we never develop a sense of gratitude and rest in our lives. Here are some examples of toxic comparison poisons and ways to fight them:

The Poison: Feeling That We're Perpetually Lacking Things
If we're always focused on what we don't have, we miss out on enjoying what we do have. This can be financially toxic for us as well as keeping us in a state of anxiety or depression related to our perceived inadequacy.

The Antidote: Developing a Gratitude Practice
When we're caught up in comparing our lives to other people's, we forget to take the time to truly appreciate what we do have. My favorite way to keep my mind occupied with gratitude is to speak thankfulness out loud around my children for the things that are easy to take for granted.

- "I feel so thankful for our warm, cozy beds and morning snuggles."
- "I love that we live so close to the L train and can hop our way into the city whenever we want to."
- "I'm so grateful to the farmers who harvested these vegetables so that we can eat this delicious dinner."

When we intentionally offer awareness toward what we have, we become more grounded in our lives and less tethered to the lives we think we should have.

The Poison: Feeling That Our Children Are Perpetually Lacking Things

When we compare our children to other people's and believe that ours are lacking, we can end up sending a message to our kids that they're not good enough. This can be about anything, including their grades, their bodies, their hobbies, or the time they spend socializing.

The Antidote: Trusting Their Process

No two kids develop in the exact same way or on the same timeline. Not even identical twins! Our job is to keep our eyes on our prizes—our children—and not let other kids' developments or achievements infect our trust in our children's unique stories. When we notice a child is different from ours and our anxiety gets triggered, we can tell ourselves, *"I can't give my child what they need if I'm trying to push them toward being something I think they should be but are not right now."*

Remember that raising secure children is not about raising children who are better than others or more accomplished. It's about raising children who have a deep sense that they're adored for exactly who they are, even when they're struggling or seemingly behind their peers.

The Poison: Putting Our Worth into Our Status

Whether we're comparing our social media numbers, waistlines, bank accounts, habitats, or achievements, it's incredibly dangerous to place our sense of our worth into the comparison blender. By judging our worth on how we compare to others, we automatically put ourselves into a pickle, because there will always be someone whose biceps are bigger, whose career is progressing faster, or who has more influence or status than we do.

The Antidote: Processing Our Attachment History

If we struggle to feel worthy, we likely had insecure dynamics within our family growing up.

Our humanity makes us worthy of belonging and connection, but if we didn't have secure attachments growing up, we may not have felt worthy of connection. This can lead us to make the mistake of believing that status makes us more worthy. While our worth cannot increase or decrease, *our sense of worth* can expand through authentic connection and the healing of early attachment wounds.

The Joneses vs Authentic Relationships

If we notice things that other people have or do that could benefit our lives, it's totally okay to use those pieces of information for learning and growing. But that never ever means using those pieces of information to put ourselves or our children down, or to forgo our core values and life goals. Remember that it's impossible to keep up with the Joneses and stay authentically connected to ourselves and our children.

If you find yourself distracted by what other people are doing or have, take some time to write out a personal mission and values statement to remind you what actually matters to you. For instance you might see a neighbor buying a new car and think, "Wow, it would be great to have that cool of a ride," but on your values list, you have, "creating a life that's debt-free and financially sustainable." Instead of feeling like you're missing out on the cool car, remind yourself that you're making an intentional life choice that's well worth the benefit of not being stressed out of your mind about car payments.

The Challenge: Ban These Comparison Contraband

These habits can keep us stuck in a comparison habit, so best to work on kicking them out of our heads as soon as they come knocking into our awareness:

- Caring more about our status in the eyes of onlookers than about our adherence to our values and our impact on our children
- Following accounts on social media that encourage us to want more, more, more, or feel less, less, less
- Validating our choices only if they mirror someone else's
- Trying to keep up with the Joneses instead of staying focused on what truly matters to us
- Using other people's successes as weapons against ourselves
- Viewing ourselves as inadequate because we're different or have different things

Compassionate Self-Talk Scripts

- *"I'm worthy of safety, belonging, and fulfillment exactly as I am. I don't need to be or have anything different to deserve these important things in my life."*
- *"I'm enough and do not need to be constantly seeking more. More is not always better. More can mean more work and more distraction. More is better when it's more gratitude, mindfulness, and connection with the people who matter the most to me."*

- *"Comparison is always bad math because there's no way to fully understand what someone else has gone through or is going through."*
- *"I have everything I need to be worthy, because worthiness is a human birthright."*

> ***Trusty Tidbit***
> **EYES ON THE PRIZE**
>
> All of my kids are on the swim team, and one of the most important skills they must develop, even before they fully master a stroke, is to learn to keep their eyes focused on the end of the lane, not on the other swimmers in the pool.
>
> If we spend too much time looking to the side (how do I measure up to the other swimmers?), we slow ourselves down.
>
> Next time you catch yourself looking sideways at someone else's swim, remember your best swim involves staying in your lane and keeping your head forward, focused on your destination, not your competition. Especially since parenting, unlike swimming, does not come with a trophy.

Further Reading

I'm Happy for You (Sort Of . . . Not Really): Finding Contentment in a Culture of Comparison by Kay Wills Wyma
The Let Them Theory by Mel Robbins
Emotional Clutter by T.K. Coleman
Love People, Use Things: Because the Opposite Never Works by Joshua Fields Millburn and Ryan Nicodemus
Validation Is for Parking: How Women Can Beat the Confidence Con by Nicole Kalil
We Can Do Hard Things by Amanda Doyle, Glennon Doyle, and Abby Wambach

How to Deal with a Denial Habit

"Denial is the way people handle what they cannot handle."

—**SHANNON ADLER**, *The Narcissistic Abuse Recovery Bible*

Denial is a defense mechanism that pops up in our lives when we feel emotionally paralyzed by a painful, scary, or uncomfortable reality that we're facing. Rather than confronting that reality, denial offers us an *alternative story* about what's happening, albeit a false story, that feels easier for us to accept.

Denial looks like:

- Focusing quickly on the bright side when something painful is happening to us or around us
- Avoiding talking about problems that are uncomfortable or unsolved
- Feeling more upset at the people bringing attention to the problems than at the people who are actively causing the problems or the problems themselves

When we struggle with denial, it's usually a result of facing trauma in our childhoods without reliable adults to help us through it. Focusing our attention away from something painful and pretending that *everything is great* is a psychologically effective way for a child stuck in a scary or uncomfortable situation to stay as calm as possible.

In that sense, denial can be helpful. It can allow us to "keep it together" until we can get to people or places that are safe enough to begin processing what happened. Sometimes things are bad enough that if we faced them in the moment, we would fall apart and lose the motivation we need to keep moving forward and through.

Denial becomes a problem however when we rely on it in adulthood. And even more so in parenthood.

If denial were a drug it would be morphine. It does nothing to help us get better; it just reduces the pain from whatever it is we are dying from, hoping that the virus goes away on its own.

How Does Our Denial Affect Our Children?

I first met Lauren when she was fresh out of an inpatient eating disorder treatment program, where she was being treated for being severely underweight. The program helped her realize that her starvation and self-denial behaviors were directly connected to a trauma that had happened to her years earlier. She had been repeatedly sexually abused by her older brother.

The abuse had lasted for a few years between the ages of around three and six. When she grew old enough to speak up for herself and recognize that something about the "play" was suspicious, the abuse had already stopped happening. She remembers thinking there was no way she could tell her parents and that the best thing to do was to tell herself, "It never happened."

Denial is an incredibly common coping response among people who have survived childhood sexual abuse, especially when the abuse occurs at the hands of a family member or close family friend. Lauren knew her parents avoided uncomfortable topics and that she often got into trouble for doing "wrong" things. Keeping this secret to herself and pretending that she'd made it up and it had never really happened felt like the natural choice.

But her body still remembered. Feelings of disgust, fear, shame, and confusion continued to flash through her head when she accidentally ended up alone in a room with her brother. She would feel panic and then shame. When she went through adolescence, the terror and confusion about her developing body and feelings overwhelmed her. She did everything she could to stop the feelings: alcohol, drugs, and eventually the sense of control she felt when she restricted herself from eating.

When she finally disclosed her experiences of abuse with her parents, they were shocked and confused. As we can all understand, this information was deeply disturbing and complex for them to process as parents.

Unfortunately for Lauren, her parents had not dealt with their own denial patterns. Rather than believing their daughter and recognizing the courage it took for her to share this trauma, they questioned her memory. ("Are you sure that's what he was doing?" "We never left you two home alone together." "Why would he do that? He was too young to know about anything sexual.")

Lauren was re-traumatized by their denial response and felt both surprised and validated by it. She recognized that perhaps the reason she'd never shared with her parents up until this point was that, on some level, she had known even as a child that denial would be their response to such a horrific situation.

Lauren realized that she had developed her denial skills by watching her parents use them. Courageously she decided that she was not interested in continuing to pretend and going back to "normal" anymore.

She let her family know that it wasn't a question of whether or not the abuse occurred and that she wouldn't be able to continue her relationship with them until they were able to address their denial and accept her truth.

Lauren's parents could no longer rely on the denial pattern they'd used their whole lives and wisely took that opportunity to go to therapy themselves. Therapy helped them both realize they had their own traumas to face and process. They had run as fast as they could from painful dynamics in their childhoods, hoping that if they just kept looking forward, nothing bad would befall their children. But in running away from their pain, they had unconsciously handed down that legacy to their children.

They came to realize that for Lauren to heal from the abuse she'd experienced, she had to acknowledge its existence. And to heal their relationships with their daughter, they had to acknowledge the ways their avoidance of uncomfortable things had made it feel scary and unnatural for her to tell them about the abuse that was happening inside their home. (And their son too, who, it turned out, had also experienced sexual abuse at an early age at the hands of a family friend.)

Let's Grow!

When we're working to deny a denial habit, our primary goals lie in growing our capacity for feeling the hard feelings while staying connected with other people.

The keys to kicking a denial habit are:

1. Learning how to feel our feelings. By tolerating what we feel and noticing that we can handle our emotional states, we're less dependent on denying what we're experiencing. (Great news—every topic in Section I: The Feelings will help you toward achieving that goal!) The more we embrace our emotions, even the negative ones, the less we have to rely on denial to cope. We discover instead that we can handle hard things and so can many of our important relationships.
2. Talking honestly about our struggles with safe people. The more we make vulnerable sharing part of our self-care routine, the less appealing denial is. We discover that being messy and having issues are the very cards we need to carry to belong with our fellow humans. And that many people want to support us and make a difference in our lives, just as we want to do in theirs.
3. Cherishing the authentic gifts of living an honest life. There's treasure and freedom in being real about the good, the bad, and the ugly in our lives. It makes us real people with real lives. Real lives are hard and complex. People who claim to never have problems are harder to relate to because they're not telling their truest truths. Radical honesty feels scary at first, but as time goes on, we learn that the scarier choice is to miss out on the deep joy that comes from having authentic relationships.

Compassionate Self-Talk Scripts

- *"Hard things are part of life, and I can acknowledge and accept them and still feel hopeful about the future."*
- *"The best stories in life involve overcoming challenges. The fact that I'm facing something hard doesn't mean I'm failing, it means I have an opportunity to do something truly meaningful."*

- *"When I feel overwhelmed by something scary, I can lean on other people for support to help get me through. I can handle hard things because I don't have to handle them in isolation."*

> ***Trusty Tidbit***
>
> **THE WISH TRICK**
>
> When we're facing painful things that we wish weren't true, and we're feeling the old itch to deny ours or someone else's reality, we can instead turn our instinct to deny into an honest wish.
>
> "I wish this wasn't happening."
> "I wish this were different."
> "I wish something else were true."
>
> Wishing is a helpful stepping stone toward feeling our grief and pain. It feels less scary somehow. The wishes we make about the painful realities in our lives help us to unlock our honest fears and tears so that we can face them more fully.

Further Reading

Am I Lying to Myself: How to Overcome Denial and See the Truth by Jane Greer, PhD

Denial: Self-Deception, False Beliefs, and the Origins of the Human Mind by Ajit Varki and Danny Brower

The Lies We Tell Ourselves: How to Face the Truth, Accept Yourself, and Create a Better Life by Jon Frederickson

How to Deal with a Distraction Habit

"Our collapsing ability to pay attention is not primarily a personal failing on my part, or your part, or your kid's part. This is being done to us all. It is being done by very powerful forces."

—JOHANN HARI, *Stolen Focus*

Sometimes I fantasize about buying a farm and spending my days tending only to my crops and my children. There are no emails, tablets, or complicated neighborhood dynamics in this fantasy. It's just me, the land, my people, and an overabundance of blackberry pies. Oh, and a porch swing. And chickens that lay fresh eggs for me every day.

It's a nice farm fantasy. Until I remember that I don't love working in the yard, or the potential failed crops, or eating the same things over and over again. And I love so many things about modern life, including reliable internet, ample running water, and accessibility to restaurants and my friends.

It isn't really modern life I don't love; it's the feeling of being pulled in so many directions that I often feel distracted from the actual moment I'm in. The farm fantasy isn't about farming; it's about simplicity and ease of presence.

Struggling with distractions in modern life is another issue discussed in this book that's par for the course for *all* parents. Even parents on farms. (That's why my vision is a fantasy and not a reality.) Being distracted, even on a daily basis, is completely normal and not a barrier to having positive relationships with our children.

A chronic distraction as a habit, however, can cause distance in our relationships with our children. It can prevent us from creating the emotional attunement and presence our kids need from us in order to cultivate feelings of deep belonging and trust.

How Does Our Chronic Distraction Affect Our Children?

When we're rarely or never able to give our children our full, undivided attention, particularly in moments when they reach out to us for support or ask us to join them in something celebratory or important to them, our distraction becomes a painful message: *you're not a priority to me.*

Of course this is rarely the reason we're distracted from our children. We're chronically distracted because we feel overwhelmed or we're doing things we think will benefit them. But even if our intention is to care for our children and keep a roof over their heads, the impact of chronic distraction on our relationships with them is profound disconnection. Eventually they stop seeking attention from us and find it elsewhere.

Let's Grow!

The best way to deal with a distraction pattern is to prioritize and protect situations in which we can be fully present. This doesn't have to require a huge effort. I like to think of presence as a juice concentrate. We don't need much to make a cup of secure relationship—just enough to flavor the relationship with a sense of overall connectedness.

Practice Protecting Presence

I find the most effective way to ensure that I'm not stuck in a chronically distracted mode is to create an *attention structure* for myself. This means I follow these simple rules to make sure I'm paying enough attention:

1. I communicate clearly when I'm able to be "all the way here" versus when I'm multitasking and unable to be fully present.
2. I give unadulterated attention during specific activities, such as family dinners, reading, and bedtime.
3. I work to use my phone as a tool and don't let myself become a tool of my phone. I do this by putting my phone away when I'm not dealing with something urgent and my kids are home, and keeping it away from my bed at night to ensure I'm not missing sleep because of the scrolling gremlins.
4. I make sure I pause if something's distracting me and ask my kids to help me eliminate its presence, so they know that I'm working to stay present.

Our children understand that life is complicated and that we're juggling many things. It's okay that we're not fully engaged with them twenty-four seven. It's about ensuring the distracted energy doesn't invade sacred times and spaces. If we're distracted all the time, our children learn to stop looking for our full presence; a true loss for both us and them.

Compassionate Self-Talk Scripts

- *"There's no greater opportunity in our lives than the chance to witness and support our children as they grow up."*
- *"A little bit of presence every day goes a long way."*
- *"Full, undivided attention is regulation pixie dust for me and my kids."*
- *"I can't be present twenty-four seven, but I can keep my eyes and ears open for the tenderness and excitement so that I can show up when it matters most."*

A NOTE ON DISTRACTEDNESS AND NEURODIVERGENCE

I would be remiss in this section not to mention that attention deficit hyperactivity disorder is a real neurological condition that can affect our ability to implement these practices for protecting presence. If you've tried repeatedly to follow these principles but find yourself unable to harness your attention, you might have a neurodivergent brain. In this case, I recommend that you research the topic and meet with a psychologist or doctor to get an assessment for a potential diagnosis and treatment.

Trusty Tidbit
SCHEDULING PRESENCE

There are so many obligations and distractions in our lives that compete for time on our calendars that it's easy to lose any unstructured time for simply being with our children in the ways they ask.

One of my favorite solutions is to schedule large blocks of sacred "off time" throughout the week that I treat with the same respect as any other priority on my calendar.

I don't fill the time or shift the time unless absolutely necessary.

When we protect time for being together without an agenda, our children can feel that our relationship with them is a priority for us, and it helps keep our attention on them and away from all the other magnetic pulls in our lives. Just as we ignore our phones during work meetings, we can ignore our phones or our work during the incredibly valuable time we're spending being present with our families.

Further Reading

Attention Span: A Groundbreaking Way to Restore Balance, Happiness and Productivity by Gloria Mark, PhD

Indistractable: How to Control Your Attention and Choose Your Life by Nir Eyal

Stolen Focus: Why You Can't Pay Attention by Johann Hari

The Now Habit: A Strategic Program for Overcoming Procrastination and Enjoying Guilt-Free Play by Neil Fiore, PhD

How to Deal with a Guilt-Tripping Habit

"Guilt-tripping is a manipulation tactic that often masquerades as love and virtue, making it hard to spot and even harder to address."

—JORDAN PICKELL, @JORDANPICKELLCOUNSELING

Guilt isn't *always* a bad habit. Feelings of guilt can be used as tools for reflection and guides for changes we need to make. Guilt can alert us to things we're doing, or not doing, that negatively impact others. As long as we're feeling guilty about something we have *actual control over*, and we're not swimming in the guilt or transforming it into a shame spiral (see page 129), then feeling guilty can help us improve our lives and relationships.

But guilt directed at someone else is never a good thing. And guilt directed from a parent to a child is never, ever a good thing. Because healthy guilt is an internal barometer guiding us toward our values, while guilt that is externalized and sent toward someone else is not a barometer, it's a weapon. It's an attempt to control the way someone else is feeling or acting, and therefore a way to avoid some sort of pain that we're feeling and haven't yet faced.

We have a guilt-tripping habit when we say things to our kids like:

- "After everything I've done for you, this is how you treat me?"
- "I guess I must just be a terrible person if you don't want to come visit."
- "I guess you just don't love me as much as I love you."
- "If you really appreciated me, you would do what I want you to do."
- "It's okay. You do what you want, I'll just sit here all by myself."

All these statements are intended to create negative guilt feelings in our children so they comply with our wishes. They're coercive and controlling. Sometimes our kids want different things from us, and we feel rejected, but that doesn't give us the right to try to stir up their guilt to change their minds. And even if they temporarily do what we want, ultimately, guilt trips don't work out the way we want them to—no close relationship can stand tall on a heap of guilt.

How Does a Guilt-Tripping Habit from Us Affect Our Children?

Unfortunately in many families, guilt-tripping is akin to a cultural tradition. Passed down by each generation to the next: a practice of making children feel guilty when they don't do, feel, think, or act in the same way as their parents.

If our children accept this tradition, then they usually also participate in it. They use guilt in their other close relationships as a way to garner what they want.

If our children see through it? The guilt trips will ultimately take our kids on trips far away from a trusting relationship with us.

Guilt trips isolate us from authentic connections with our children because control is the kryptonite to connection. The moment we feel obligated or trapped in a relationship, we lose our own sense of agency in that space, which dampens desire and gratitude. *It just doesn't feel good to feel bad about being ourselves in a relationship.*

The guilt-tripping instinct is activated in us when we sense that we may be becoming less central in our children's lives, either in terms of influencing their behavior or identity, or in terms of the time and commitment they spend in their relationship with us.

Guilt-tripping can be effective in persuading our children to do what we want them to do in terms of *going through the motions*, but it's wildly ineffective at creating the type of authentic connection we actually want with them.

Every time we use guilt to try to manipulate an outcome, we're eroding our children's genuine desire to be close to us. Instead of being someone whom our children can come to for support and refuge, we become a stressful place where they have to perform to avoid the discomfort of our guilt.

Examples of Guilt-Trippy Behavior

- We respond dramatically with puppy eyes or whining sounds when our children refuse affection or an invitation to spend time with us.
- We tell our children that they're *hurting us* when they take steps in directions that are contrary to what we want from them.
- We pout or take it personally when they develop close relationships with other people.

- We passive-aggressively complain about our loneliness or helplessness when our children are increasing their independence from us.
- We believe that since we spent our lives pleasing our parents, it's our turn to be pleased by our children, who should be focusing on us and not themselves.

Let's Grow!

The opposite of guilt-tripping is grief and then self-care. When we try to guilt our children into doing or feeling certain things, we're ignoring the core needs or losses that are needing our attention.

For example, let's say our children are hitting adolescence and feeling much more invested in time with their peers than time with us. This is normal. They're learning to bond with people outside of their family. It doesn't mean that they don't love or appreciate us or even want to be close to us. It means they're working on something that doesn't happen to involve us in the ways their younger developmental tasks did.

This can trigger all sorts of emotions in us. Perhaps we've not been investing in our other relationships, and our child's increased independence is activating loneliness for us. Then it's our job to head to page 78 and figure out how to deal with our loneliness instead of guilting our children into staying home on Friday night to watch *Gilmore Girls* while their friends go to the football game.

Or perhaps we're worried about them going out with their friends because we don't want anything traumatic to happen to them. Especially if something happened to us when we were their age. This indicates we have trauma that needs tending, and instead of trying to guilt them into staying home so we can feel less worried, we need to figure out how to deal with our trauma (see page 142) and work through that worry in a way that doesn't stifle their independence.

Whenever we feel the urge to take our kids on a guilt trip, we need to pause and take ourselves on a growth trip instead.

To keep ourselves away from this bad habit, remember these three things about guilt:

1. Guilt can be a helper when it's *felt internally* and related to something we *can* change.
2. Guilt can be a weapon when it's *launched externally* and we use it to try to get someone else to do what we want.
3. Guilt can be a highlighter for the care that we need.

Compassionate Self-Talk Scripts

- *"It's normal to feel sad when my kids are gaining independence, but that doesn't mean it's their job to stop launching or to care for my feelings about it."*
- *"When I feel the urge to send guilt toward my child, I should take some time to be curious about what I'm needing instead."*
- *"My children don't owe me anything. I, however, do owe them the effort of taking care of myself when I'm struggling with the reality that they're separate beings and not always going to do or feel what I hope they will."*

Trusty Tidbit
DEBT FORGIVENESS

When I was in the eighth grade, my mom took me out for a special dinner and unforgettable conversation at Healthy Habits salad bar (rest in peace HH).

After we finished eating she pulled out a box and a note. In the box was a necklace with a rose on it that she said she wanted me to wear to remind me that watching me grow had been a beautiful experience for her.

In the note was a message that simply said, "You don't ever owe me anything. Being your mother has been one of my life's greatest joys and is not a debt you ever have to repay."

!!!!!!!!! Even as an angsty early adolescent, I knew this was a sacred gift. And here we are, thirty years later, and she has kept to that mentality.

And guess what? I will fight anyone I have to for the honor of getting to care for her in her aging. I won't do it because I have to, I'll do it because I'll feel the same honor changing her diapers as she felt changing mine.

Further Reading

Break the Cycle: A Guide to Healing Intergenerational Trauma by Dr. Mariel Burqué

Emotional Blackmail: When the People in Your Life Use Fear, Obligation, and Guilt to Manipulate You by Dr. Susan Forward and Donna Frazier

The Highly Sensitive Person's Guide to Dealing with Toxic People by Shahida Arabi

Transform Your Guilt and Shame: Evidence-Based Strategies to Heal from Trauma and Adversity by Carolyn B. Allard

How to Deal with a

Numbing Habit

"The thing you want offers relief, but it's a trap."

—**TESS CALLAHAN**, *April and Oliver*

If we didn't have parents who could help us navigate our emotions growing up, we naturally had to find alternative ways to cope. When we're not born into the good fortune of having a *calm*, emotionally present parent, then we ultimately rely on the sustenance of *numbness* that anything else can offer.

Emotional pain without support is excruciating and intolerable. Especially when we're children and our brains are still developing the capacity to process emotions. Most of us who have a numbing habit developed it when we were young. We learned that the best way to address our pain was to find a way to *stop feeling it*. We didn't have anyone who could teach us that pain can be released and processed.

We developed numbing habits that offered us *relief* instead of *regulation or healing*. These include:

- Emotional eating
- Frequent use of legal or illegal drugs or alcohol
- Scrolling the internet
- Excessive shopping
- Reckless gambling
- Obsessive exercising
- Anxious cleaning
- Being perpetually busy
- Compulsive sexual behavior
- Binge-watching television
- Fixating on work

These habits never give us what we actually need. Instead of making us more fulfilled and whole, these habits keep us in a cycle of craving and numbing. Despite an awareness that they're causing us harm, we continue to repeat the behaviors. The harm might be to our physical health, our financial stability, or, as is most common, to our relationships with the people closest to us. And most sadly, to our children who need us to help them regulate *their* emotional pain so they don't have to turn toward numbing as well.

How Does Our Numbing Habit Affect Our Children?

When we numb to cope, we also disappear. We might not disappear entirely. We might be technically in the room, or even coherent enough to know what's happening, but we've disconnected the parts of ourselves that offer emotional availability and presence to our children.

Our kids may not understand why we feel absent or "sort of gone," but they can tell that we are not fully online. And most kids blame themselves for our distance, assuming they've done something to make us shut down or go away.

Our numbing habits create distance, and they create models. When we numb ourselves as a habit, our children witness it. Even if they don't see the exact thing we do, they know something's happening to take us into an altered state. The degree to which our numbing affects our children is, of course, related to the degree of absence our numbing habits create.

Let's Grow!

The steps we need to take to address a numbing habit vary significantly depending on the severity of our habit. How we address a numbing habit depends on what tactics we've been using to numb ourselves and how long we've been engaged in that particular coping pattern.

How to Deal with a Mild to Moderate Numbing Habit

If you're aware that you're engaging in numbing habits that you want to stop, and you're fairly positive that you can, that's fantastic! I love it when that happens.

Step 1: Acknowledge the numbing pattern you want to stop.

Step 2: Make this acknowledgment official by sharing it with two to three people.

Step 3: Identify the feelings or situations that you are numbing away from.

Step 4: Work on increasing your ability to tolerate those feelings and situations by increasing the amount of support you have in dealing with them.

Step 5: Work on creating positive relational and mindfulness habits that replace the numbing habits and increase your connectedness to others.

Rinse and repeat. As many times as you need to. Forever. Some habits need us to break them repeatedly until they finally lose their grip on our brains and bodies. Keep trying. You got this.

How to Deal with a Numbing Habit That's Probably an Addiction

Before I start defining an addiction, I want to say something very loudly and clearly. ADDICTION IS NOT A MORAL FAILURE. I'm sorry for the capital letters, I just needed to make sure I was louder than the incredible volume of shame and cruelty that's often hurled at anyone in the grips of an addiction.

Addiction is a neurological brain pattern that's incredibly challenging to circumvent. It can lead to terrible choices, no doubt. But the shame and stigma associated with addiction are extremely unhelpful in the quest to escape it. We don't address an addiction problem by shaming ourselves or someone else. We address it by truly understanding what it is and how we can loosen its grip on our bodies and lives.

And. As someone who loves many, many, many, many, many, (did I say many?) family members, friends, and clients who have battled or are battling addiction, I know personally the devastation and pain that can come from being caught in its inevitable crossfire. So if you're in a place where you find it hard to feel compassionate toward yourself or someone you know who's struggling with addiction, I see you. It is hard to stay compassionate when the wreckage is so profound. It took me a long time to release my resentment toward my dad's addiction to alcohol and to recognize that shame was a barrier to his recovery.

Because if we believe that addiction is shameful or amoral, or that someone has a "choice" to simply stop, then the person with the addiction often becomes more defensive and isolated. Instead, when we say, “Addiction is an awful experience that people get caught in and need help getting out of,” it offers us a far more dignified route to getting help.

If you have a twinge that you might be battling addiction, I hope you’ll keep reading even if it triggers shame or panic from that stupid stigma we’re still working to dispel.

I define addiction as *a chronic, compulsive drive to consume something for temporary feelings of pleasure or relief, despite the severe and enduring negative consequences or harm it causes in our lives and the lives of the people around us.*

We can be addicted to *substances* such as alcohol or cocaine, and we can be addicted to *activities* that encourage substance production (primarily dopamine) in our brains, including gambling and pornography. While these addictions have different implications and negative effects, they all affect our ability to be secure and reliable attachment figures. Why? Because they orient us to prioritize the addiction over our well-being and to reduce our literal and emotional availability for our children.

Signs that we have an addiction we need to deal with include:

- Our actions related to a substance or an activity have caused harm to people we love, but we’ve not been able to stop despite feeling ashamed and guilt-ridden.
- Our friends or family have communicated concerns to us about our habit.
- We lack motivation to do things we previously enjoyed and only want the substance or activity.
- We’re preoccupied with our next encounter with the addictive substance or activity and think about it throughout our day.
- The longer we use the substance or activity, the larger our mood swings and the more frequently we’re irritable or angry.

- Our life begins to revolve around our craving for the substance or activity.
- We frequently downplay our use or lie about it to people we care about.

Confessing that we have a problem with addiction is not admitting that we are a problem, or even that we intentionally caused one. It's just saying that we're in water we don't know how to get out of, and we need some buoys and search lights to help us get to shore.

Once we've recognized that we have an addiction to work through, the next step is figuring out who can help. We should never try to "white knuckle" an addiction on our own. Stopping substance use without evaluation is dangerous, and in the case of alcohol use, can lead to seizures and even death.

How Do You Find Help?

My favorite thing to tell someone who wants to start a recovery process is: look for other people around you already on the path. Who do you know who has already sought out help for their addictions? Who do you trust to understand the complexity you're feeling and facing without judgment or condescension? Ask those folks where they started and who they know and trust in the recovery community.

If you don't know anyone in recovery, or anyone you feel comfortable reaching out to, there are free in-person support groups, such as Alcoholics Anonymous and Narcotics Anonymous, as well as many online support groups. If those groups give you the heebie-jeebies for whatever reason, google community resources such as mental health centers or community counseling groups that offer individual and group support for anyone wanting to recover from addiction.

Chances are it will take you a few attempts to find the people and help that feel right for you. That's normal. It's important you don't give up and you keep looking for people who get you, get your situation, and can help you figure out a path forward.

You are absolutely, positively not alone. Millions upon millions of people battle addictions, and though not everyone goes into recovery, millions of people do.

Trusty Tidbit

INCREASE CONNECTION TO DECREASE ADDICTION

The opposite of addiction isn't sobriety, although sobriety is usually an essential step toward recovery. The opposite of addiction is a secure connection. Addictions develop when we don't have other people to help co-regulate us. Instead of using relationships to help us feel safe and calm, we turn to substances. Unfortunately those substances offer us temporary refuge from the pain in our lives, but they don't take away the issues causing that pain. Especially emotional isolation.

The first step toward recovering from addiction is finding people who can support us along our journeys to learn how to feel safe without our numbing habits.

This is why Alcoholics Anonymous and other group-oriented recovery programs are so successful in my opinion. Because to refrain from addictions, we need authentic belonging and support.

Compassionate Self-Talk Scripts

- *"My numbing habit is a coping pattern I no longer need. I'm capable of facing my feelings and finding safe people to feel them with."*
- *"Even if I chose numb over connection in the past, that doesn't mean I can't change the present and the future."*
- *"My feelings are not liabilities; they're helpers guiding me toward the support I need to find."*
- *"I am not my addiction."*
- *"I can take a small step today to start my recovery journey."*

Further Reading

Beyond Addiction: How Science and Kindness Help People Change by Jeffrey Foote

Blackout: Remembering the Things I Drank to Forget by Sarah Hepola

In the Realm of Hungry Ghosts by Gabor Maté, foreword by Peter Levine

Never Enough: The Neuroscience and Experience of Addiction by Judith Grisel

Quit Like a Woman: The Radical Choice to Not Drink in a Culture Obsessed with Alcohol by Holly Whitaker

STUMBLES AND STEPS

My younger brother was ten years old when he had his first alcoholic beverage. Not a taste of an alcoholic beverage, a grown-up quantity of one. He wasn't simply being curious either. He wanted to find a way to disappear. He was a neurodivergent kid drowning in big *T* trauma without any idea of how to get ashore. How he felt when he drank relieved him of how he felt when he was sober. So he started to chase the feeling of not feeling.

Unfortunately alcoholism runs rampant in our family tree, and he inherited the genetic predisposition for addiction. He also inherited the family tradition of staying functional enough to deny the addiction. He could achieve enough in his life to convince himself that the only problem was other people thinking he had a problem.

If you had asked me a few years back if I thought he would ever change or recover, I would have given you a confident "not likely." I spent decades trying to help him recognize the self-destructive patterns I saw him going through. For almost thirty years his cycle looked like this:

1. Drink a lot and often
2. Get scared by something that he did or by something that happened to him while he was drunk
3. Stop drinking (to convince himself it wasn't a drinking problem)
4. Feel better
5. Start drinking again
6. Repeat from step one

I felt a responsibility to help him get healthy until I finally realized that was unhealthy for me. I was acting out of codependence and not accepting the reality that he didn't want my help. So I stopped helping, which was one of the hardest jobs I've ever had to quit. Not because I ever wanted the job, but because I was so afraid that if I gave up, I would lose him forever.

And being honest, it did mean that I lost him. The more I took care of myself, the less capable I was of trying to rescue him in steps two and three of his cycle or to pretend with him in steps one, four, and five. The less capable I was of being enmeshed with his addiction cycle, the less we were in each other's lives in any meaningful way.

Until . . .

He hit a stumble a couple of years ago that shook him to his core. Folks in the recovery community would call this a "rock bottom." His marriage ended, and his sense of his place in the world right alongside it. He was devastated and bewildered. And ready to take a step outside of his addiction cycle. I'll never forget the night he called me and was at the brink of giving up completely. He couldn't see the value of his life anymore. I rushed over to his house and, after consoling him and a few hours of sobering up, he said to me, "I don't think I can drink anymore."

That was the first step. Just saying it out loud to himself and to me. Acknowledging that he didn't feel in control of the drinking or his life and that if he was being completely honest, he never had.

That step led to other steps, which have led to a long walk into sobriety and some really beautiful changes in his life. One day at a time, he has slowly moved into a very different relationship with his children, himself, and everyone else in the world. Losing my brother for that long was truly sad, but gaining him now? It's a gift I don't think I could have fully appreciated if I'd never lost him in the first place.

We walk back into people's hearts and lives not with grand gestures or promises, but with courageous self-reflection and the effort it takes to walk step-by-step toward recovery and health.

How to Deal with an Over-Protective Rescue Habit

"Sweater, n. Garment worn by a child when its mother is feeling chilly."

—**AMBROSE BIERCE**, *The Unabridged Devil's Dictionary*

It is absolutely normal and essential that we do what we can to protect our children from *serious harm.* It's a huge part of our hero role. When we can protect our children in truly dangerous situations in which they're not yet capable of protecting themselves, it's a blessing in their lives and ours.

But there's a difference between responding to real threats in our environment and holding an overprotective rescue mindset in which we prevent our children from taking any risks, facing natural consequences, or learning how to tolerate normal painful feelings.

When we believe, "*It's my job to make sure my child never feels discomfort or pain,*" we will inevitably develop an overprotective habit. An overprotective habit is a compulsion in response to the pressure and anxiety that earlier beliefs trigger in our bodies (also see How to Deal with Feeling Anxious, page 21).

We have an overprotective rescue mindset if:

- We hold a level of anxiety that keeps us hypervigilant and always on guard concerning our children (or anyone else we feel responsible for).
- We confuse our children's discomfort (normal emotional responses to life) with trauma.
- We try to arrange ourselves and our world to prevent any discomfort for our children.
- We jump in between our children and potential mistakes or rejections to fix things for them *before* they face consequences or losses.
- We feel guilty and harshly blame ourselves when our children experience pain.

I've found that this habit develops for one of two reasons:

1. We grew up in a family where this mindset was present and normalized, and we adopted it internally without even realizing it was overprotective. It feels normal to us.
2. We grew up in a family where we felt a painful lack of protection and have sworn to never let our children feel unprotected as we did. We don't know what feels normal, but we don't want our painful experiences to be passed on to our kids.

In either of those situations, we didn't experience what secure relating looks like. We didn't learn that feelings need to be felt, and that feeling feelings with people who care about us is much more tolerable than feeling feelings in isolation.

We learned that feeling alone in our pain or worry was *awful*, and to be terrified of feeling pain because our parents couldn't handle it. Now we're trying to prevent our children from feeling pain by constantly helicoptering over them.

How Does an Overprotective Rescue Habit Affect Our Children?

Unfortunately, this approach creates a repellent effect that causes our children to find our presence intrusive and overbearing and to hide information from us to increase their independence. The lived experience of an overprotected child isn't "I feel protected," it's "I feel that my parents don't trust me to handle things," or that pain and suffering is catastrophic and can't be navigated.

When we constantly rescue our children from discomfort, pain, failure, or rejection, we also deny them the opportunity to develop grit, resilience, and trust in our ability to be there for them during the inevitable hard seasons of life.

Overprotecting and rescuing can leave our children without the emotional support and life experience they need to feel secure in life and to feel confident that they can rely on us when things are hard.

Let's Grow!

If we want our children to feel secure with us and to come to us for support when they're struggling, we need to learn to do these three things:

- Regulate our anxiety by changing our beliefs about our role in our children's relationships to pain and struggle.
- Accurately attune to their emotional states. If you struggle with this, find a friend who seems to be comfortable talking about feelings. Plan a regular call with them and ask them to help you notice, tolerate, and talk about emotions. Developing awareness of your own emotions will help you recognize them in your children more easily.

- Learn how to tolerate our feelings that arise in the presence of our child's emotional pain.

Our kids need to know that we can handle our painful feelings (by seeing us calm ourselves when we get worked up or worried), and they need to know that we can handle *their* emotional states (by seeing us stay present and emotionally grounded when *they* are in emotional pain).

NEURODIVERGENCE NOTE (HIGH SENSITIVITY IN PARENTS)

For those of us who are hard-wired with a particularly sensitive nervous system, it can be more challenging to let our children experience pain and struggle. We feel their feelings deeply (the same as we feel our own), so the process of standing by and not stepping in can feel like we're abandoning them.

But there's a big difference between abandoning our children to feel their pain in isolation and allowing our children to face pain with our support.

If you know that you're "a highly sensitive person," a phrase coined by the research of the incredible Elaine Aron, make sure you have a couple of trusted supports who can help you determine whether your reactions are in tune with your child or heightened because of your sensitivity. This can be hard to ascertain on your own when even subtle emotions put your nervous system on high alert.

Trusty Tidbit

PAIN PREVENTION VS ISOLATION PREVENTION

It's not our job to prevent our children from experiencing emotional pain, discomfort, or natural consequences. (This is not possible or recommended.)

It is our job to prevent our children from feeling emotionally isolated when they're experiencing emotional pain, discomfort, or natural consequences.

Resilience is not built from the absence of pain, but rather from the absence of having to handle pain without support.

No human being escapes emotional heartache, but that doesn't mean we can't make a huge difference in our children's experiences of pain and suffering.

When hard emotions show up for our kids, we can offer them the gifts of presence and understanding. We can teach them what we know about emotions.

And in turn we'll be showing them that they can securely rely on us when times are tough.

Compassionate Self-Talk Scripts

- *"It's not my job to prevent my child from experiencing pain and discomfort. It's my job to prevent my child from having to navigate pain and discomfort in isolation."*
- *"Not all struggle is trauma. I can stand by my child in their struggles and attune to their requests for support instead of constantly inserting myself in fear that they feel traumatized and can't handle it themselves."*
- *"If my child is feeling uncomfortable about something they need to do to grow, I can offer them compassion and also hold a boundary, so whatever is making them feel uncomfortable eventually becomes comfortable for them. This isn't mean, it's something they sometimes need from me."*

Further Reading

Get Out of Your Own Way: Overcoming Self-Defeating Behavior by Mark Goulston, MD, and Philip Goldberg

Hunt, Gather, Parent: What Ancient Cultures Can Teach Us About the Lost Art of Raising Children by Michaeleen Doucleff, PhD

Raising Securely Attached Kids by Eli Harwood (specifically chapter four, "Feelings Are for Feeling")

The Mountain Is You: Transforming Self-Sabotage into Self-Mastery by Brianna Wiest

The Overparenting Epidemic: Why Helicopter Parenting Is Bad for Your Kids . . . and Dangerous for You, Too! by George Glass, MD, and David Tabatsky

How to Deal with a People-Pleasing Habit

"When you say yes to others, make sure you are not saying no to yourself."

—PAULO COELHO

People-pleasing is being overly generous and gratuitous to other people out of fear that they might harm, reject, or abandon us if we don't.

When we have a problematic people-pleasing habit, we not only dote on others out of fear, we also neglect ourselves at a level that's harmful to our own well-being.

People-pleasing is a trauma response to relational experiences with caregivers or close partners who had narcissistic wounds or tendencies. At some point in our life journeys, we had to please someone to get our basic needs met (safety, shelter, and belonging). This means that we learned to silence our own needs, preferences, desires, and instincts to revolve around someone else.

A synonym for people-pleasing is "fawning," and it's considered by many in the psychological community to be part of our inborn instincts, along with the fight, flight, freeze, and faint responses. If another person, our community, or the system we live under is a source of danger (i.e., they have the intent or power to harm us in some way through abuse or neglect), we learn to please them as an attempt to reduce the harm they do to us.

STOP

If you're in a relationship with someone who makes demands and scares or punishes you when you don't comply, you may be caught in an abusive dynamic. If someone is emotionally, physically, or sexually coercing or forcing you to do things you don't want to do, please reach out to a domestic violence hotline to get specialized help from advocates who understand what you're going through.

How Does a People-Pleasing Habit Affect Our Children?

When we have a problematic people-pleasing habit, our nervous systems are stuck in a state of hypervigilance toward the perceived needs and wants of others (especially those with more narcissistic traits). This means we're not in tune with ourselves or our children (making it hard to give them gift #1, feeling that we can handle what they feel).

If we're trying to please our children, it means we're out of touch with their actual needs and are projecting onto them that they have the power to abandon or hurt us. This can get in the way

> ***Trusty Tidbit***
>
> **MAKING SACRIFICES FOR OUR KIDS ≠ SACRIFICING OURSELVES FOR THEM**
>
> There's a difference between the sacrifices we have to make on our parenting journey (sleep, finances, time, our previous lifestyles, or our images of ourselves!) and getting into a mode that causes us to forget to take care of ourselves.
>
> If we're never thinking of our needs, never taking the time to do the things we love, never saying no, or always giving, giving, giving, we're sacrificing ourselves, which doesn't benefit our children.
>
> Because we're going to become depleted, desperate, and likely resentful. When we forsake ourselves for the sake of our children, we end up getting in the way of our actual goals. Our children need us to be secure for them, and this means we must be mindful of our own physical, emotional, social, and spiritual health.
>
> Yes, make sacrifices at times when your children need you to but remember never to sacrifice yourself or your overall well-being because they need you to be healthy enough to connect with them, guide them, and model self-care for them.

of gift #2, because if we're inaccurately projecting our insecurity onto them, we can't pick up on their perspectives accurately. When we live in a people-pleasing state, our children learn two unfortunate things:

1 They can't rely on us as models of self-assurance or self-advocacy.
2 People-pleasing is normal.

Both these things put our children at risk of getting involved in lopsided or even abusive relationships. Without the skills necessary to speak up for themselves, they're likely to recreate this pattern in themselves. Or to swing wildly in the other direction.

Let's Grow!

Instead of teaching our children that it's their job to keep others satisfied or pleased, we want to model for them relationships that are based on reciprocity. Reciprocity means a dynamic in which both people are attentive and caring toward each other. The love goes both ways. The respect goes both ways. The care and curiosity and safety go both ways.

The steps to shifting from a people-pleasing mindset to a reciprocity mindset are:

1. Address Underlying Anxiety and Trauma: We usually develop a fierce people-pleasing habit because it was programmed into us via a traumatic relationship. These past experiences need healing so they don't continue to take up so much space in our present relationships. (see Feeling Traumatized on page 142)
2. Reset Responsibility Metrics: We have to allow other people to be responsible for keeping the connection healthy as much as ourselves. Which means some of our relationships will crumble. Some people won't be willing or able to care for us in the ways we care for them. If that's the case, it's probably time to say "adieu."
3. Practice Self-Advocacy: Just because we've decided to let other people shoulder more of the responsibility for the relationship, it doesn't mean that they will know automatically how to care

for us. We have to speak up clearly for what we want and need, even when it doesn't fit in with the other person's preferences. And like anything else, practice makes progress.

This is a habit that tends to shift most effectively when we get fed up with it or when we can see how it's damaging our health or affecting our children. Ideally we'll shift our self-abandoning habit long before it's taken that toll.

When I was in graduate school, I ended up in a relationship with someone who was emotionally and sexually abusive toward me. I use the term "ended up" intentionally because, as I've processed the trauma of that relationship, I've recognized how much of my people-pleasing habit was part of the dynamic even before we

Trusty Tidbit

WATCH OUT FOR THE SWINGING PENDULUM

People-pleasing is a very challenging habit to break. But once we decide to stop pleasing people, we can accidentally swing our pendulum to the other extreme.

If we swing too far in the other direction, we could go from being "all give" to being "no give."

Healthy relationships hold space for both people's needs and involve turn-taking, compromise, and mutual recognition.

Being empowered to speak our voice and be a part of a relationship doesn't mean always getting things our way or seeing all conflict as an attempt to take away our voice.

Successful recovery from people-pleasing means we're willing to bring our needs into our relationships while we also stay receptive to the needs of others.

began dating. I never really wanted to be with this person, but after politely saying no a few times, I didn't have the skills or determination to assertively displease someone who was so persuasive and determined.

Also everyone else seemed to think he was great, and other women in my cohort liked him and told me I was lucky that he was so into me. Rather than trusting my body's reactions to his pursuit of me, I abandoned myself by concluding that my hesitance was the problem and not that my feelings were being ignored and invalidated.

Long story short, the relationship was one of the most emotionally and physically painful experiences of my life. I've been through some hard stuff, but there's something particularly brutal about being demeaned and controlled by someone who tells you that they love you.

I was able to eventually leave that relationship because a brave group of friends introduced me to the power and control wheel and taught me about the cycle of intimate partner violence. Once I saw the writing on the wall, I knew I wanted to get out before I got in deeper. We weren't married and didn't have children, so leaving was simple in terms of practicalities.

But leaving someone who is desperately begging me to stay is my most vulnerable Achilles' heel. I never want anyone to feel abandoned by me. It took me some time with incredible friends and therapists to finally recognize that by staying with someone who was abusive toward me, I was actually abandoning myself. Once I could see that, I managed to free myself and spend my time and energy on the safe and secure people in my life. I sometimes think back to what would have happened if I'd stayed in that relationship, and I'm so thankful that I left. By leaving, I saved the only person in the dynamic that I could save. Myself.

It usually feels scary when we drop a people pleasing habit, but when we finally start to emerge from underneath the unhealthy edict of perpetually pleasing others, we find that life is far less disorienting and far more fun. You deserve to be a genuine part of every relationship you are in.

Compassionate Self-Talk Scripts

- *"It's not my job to make sure other people feel happy with me, it's my job to be kind to other people and expect them to be kind to me as well."*
- *"If someone is enraged when they don't feel satisfied, that doesn't mean I failed them, it means they have expectations of me that are hostile and unfair."*
- *"I'm worthy of a place at the table, and healthy, safe people will be thrilled when I take up more space with them."*

Further Reading

Codependent No More: How to Stop Controlling Others and Start Caring for Yourself by Melody Beattie

Fawning: Why The Need to Please Others Makes Us Lose Ourselves—And How To Find Our Way Back by Dr. Ingrid Clayton

Good Kids: Why You Suffered in Silence and How to Break the Cycle with Your Kids by Maggie Nick

It's Not You: Identifying and Healing from Narcissistic People by Dr. Ramani Durvasula

Set Boundaries, Find Peace: A Guide to Reclaiming Yourself by Nedra Glover Tawwab

How to Deal with a Perfectionism Habit

"What people somehow forgot to mention when we were children was that we need to make messes in order to find out who we are and why we are here."

—**ANNE LAMOTT**, *Bird by Bird*

A perfectionism habit is a really tricky booger. When we're stuck in the habit, we believe that perfectionism is helping us move toward "excellence" and "achievement," but it's actually anxiety in a fancy dress. Perfectionism keeps us running at an *unmaintainable pace* toward *unattainable performance*. It says to us, "*If you get everything right, you'll be safe, lovable, worthy, etc.*" But the perfectionistic habit always spots some way that we're imperfect, and lo and behold, we never actually reach the promised land of feeling safe, lovable, and worthy.

Perfectionism is a scam; it keeps us emotionally stuck and isolated from genuine connection.

Sometimes perfectionism is aimed only at us, but it can also spread toward our children.

Perfectionism in parenting looks like:

- We view our mistakes or our children's mistakes as failures.

- We struggle to complete tasks and procrastinate due to unrealistic expectations.
- We're highly critical of ourselves, our work, our children, our parenting, etc.
- We're highly critical of others and focus on what could have been better without ever celebrating the accomplishments and milestones.
- We have an "all or nothing" mentality about performance (second place is the first loser).
- We struggle with feedback and feel that "room for improvement" really means that we failed.
- We struggle to take risks out of fear that we'll not meet our standards.
- We fail to consider context when evaluating ourselves or our children.
- We feel acute shame and guilt when we think we've done something wrong.

How Does Our Perfectionism Habit Affect Our Children?

When we struggle with perfectionism, our children do too. Because we set the standards and expectations in our children's lives, they hear and see the incredibly high measuring stick we berate ourselves with and will come to believe that stick also belongs to them.

When perfectionism infects a family environment, it cultivates high stress and tension for our children because their development feels like a tightrope walk. They can't explore and take risks without envisioning the fall from the rope. Instead of having time to wonder and wander as they learn, they're riddled with fear that they'll fail and disappoint us or themselves.

Perfectionism also increases the chance that our children will hide their reality from us when life inevitably gets messy. If our expectations are unrealistic, either for us or for them, they'll know this and will intuitively keep their struggles and tender emotions out of our view. Behind closed doors, they'll try to "sort out" the parts of themselves they perceive as unacceptable, leaving them isolated and without care and guidance through potentially tricky life stages or events.

One of the dearest young men I've ever worked with was deeply affected by the unexamined perfectionism habit he inherited from his family growing up. Anthony came from a family that was working very hard to step out of the generational trauma of poverty. His grandparents had labored in truly heroic ways to offer his parents opportunities for higher education, and his parents had taken those opportunities and crossed every *t* and dotted every *i*.

As an African American family with a legacy of serious trauma through Jim Crow, and likely more ancestral trauma floating back to the enslavement of Black folks on plantations, the pressure to perform was based on historical survival.

Anthony knew his parents allowed themselves very little margin for error in their lives. They held incredibly strict ethics and self-discipline, and strove ceaselessly toward their goals. Because of the reality of racism, discrimination, and stereotyping, Anthony and his family were under tremendous pressure to be seen as exceptional, which meant never making a mistake.

Unfortunately, these extremely high expectations made it feel impossible for Anthony to share with his parents when he was hit with a deep and unyielding depression during his freshman year of college. Rather than calling them and being honest about his slipping grades and increasing sense of suicidal ideation, he lied to them, doubling his sense of shame and worthlessness.

Luckily Anthony had a friend who was paying attention to his decline and was courageous enough to get Anthony to my office for therapy.

Because he was so far into his depression, I had to involve his parents to ensure he was safe when he wasn't with me. He *did not* want me to call them. He was convinced they would be disappointed and angry and see his depression as a failure.

As it turned out, they were extremely grateful to get the call and to be able to show up for their son. They had also struggled in silence during their own childhoods and hadn't realized that their standards were making it hard for Anthony to be authentic with them about his inner reality.

Even though we all wished Anthony had not had to go through an excruciating depressive episode, his entire family would tell you that it was the very wake-up call they needed to realize how much pressure everyone was under and how much more room for messy feelings and honest sharing they all needed with each other.

Dealing with this habit is about learning not only to accept imperfections, but to believe they add value to our lives. When we honor the messiness of life with the people closest to us, we honor our humanity together, and that is how we make belonging soup.

Let's Grow!

Perfectionism can feel impossible to quit when it's been such a reliable coping mechanism for so long, but it can be done! By naming it for what it is, we can see it as a problem and not a solution. Then we can practice allowing ourselves to experience failures, which then connects us more authentically to other people. When we discover that it's our humanness that bonds us together, it becomes far easier to release the reins on perfectionism.

> ***Trusty Tidbit***
>
> **PARENTING IS GRADED ON A CURVE**
>
> I want to reassure all of us that the research on the parent-child relationship has given us comforting data showing that the number of parents who can cultivate secure relationships is not remotely close to 100 percent. We've found that secure parents are positively connected with children around 30–50 percent of the time! This assignment is too hard for anyone to ace because parent-child relationships involve so much complexity and nuance.
>
> According to psychologist DW Winnicott, a "good enough" parent is one who is regulated enough, supportive enough, and available enough.
>
> So please don't panic when you get negative feedback on your parenting assignment. The secure parenting process allows for quite a few wrong answers to pass the test. Not to mention that your children bringing negative feedback to your attention is a sign they trust you to hear them, care about their feelings, and to respond safely and maturely. That's some generational success to be sure.

Call It Out, Stall It Out

When we acknowledge that we struggle with perfectionism with the people we trust and care about, we take a huge leap away from the habit. Why? Because to say that we struggle with perfectionism is to say that we struggle. That we're not perfect. And when we do that with trusted people, we discover that we feel more loved, not less.

Detailing with other people the pressured standards that we hold for ourselves and our children can help us recognize the harm in those standards. It can feel embarrassing at first to open up about the measuring sticks we've been using to beat ourselves with, but it gives us a chance to receive validation from others that these standards are not reasonable or healthy for anyone.

Aim to Fail

If you've been locked in a perfectionism mindset for a long time, my guess is that you've worked very hard not to let yourself "fail" at anything. The anxiety inherent in the mentality has led you to believe that you can't handle failure and that it will be the absolutely worst, most painful thing ever.

But failure is simply a part of life and learning. It happens to everyone. And when we discover that we can recover from failure, it helps us to evolve and take more risks. This is how human beings develop best. With opportunities to try new things, fail at them, and learn something new as a result. Then to either try again or try something else.

If this feels overwhelmingly scary, start with little things. If you've never tried painting or knitting, take a stab at it even if you know your first attempts will look like kindergarten projects. Try a new recipe that's out of your comfort zone and relax while you do it, let it cook a little too long, or put in a little too much butter (this is a personal life hack). Notice that even if the soufflé doesn't poof, you've not lost any value as a person, and it might even still taste good.

Turn Up the Vulnerability Volume

Underneath a perfectionism mindset is a deeply embedded fear that we're not worthy of belonging and connection. And a mistaken belief that if we clean ourselves up enough, we can somehow turn the volume up on our worthiness. But we can't increase our worthiness for belonging and connection, we can only turn up our *sense* of worthiness. And the data is clear—that doesn't happen by having it all together. It happens by being vulnerable and authentic with the safe and loving people in our lives.

If this is especially challenging for you, it could be helpful to join a support group or set a daily alarm on your phone that says, "Have you let anyone see the messy sides of your life today?" and then notice how those connections grow as a result. We feel closest to people who trust us with their vulnerable truths because that's how intimacy is born.

Compassionate Self-Talk Scripts

- *"Struggling is a part of the human journey and not a reflection of my worthiness for connection or belonging."*
- *"The pressure I feel to be perfect is the voice of anxiety or past trauma, not an accurate message about who I need to be or how I need to do things."*
- *"My flaws and flubs are opportunities for vulnerability and increased closeness in my relationships. It is when we share ourselves authentically that our deepest bonds are formed."*

Trusty Tidbit

WHEN ACHIEVEMENTS GET IN THE WAY OF CONFIDENCE

When we're stuck in a perfectionism habit, achievement becomes our drug. We constantly seek to be, have, perform, or appear in ways that alleviate our anxiety. If only I am . . . , then I'll be acceptable, lovable, or worthy.

When this happens in our lives, no achievement is enough, which means our achievements perpetuate our anxiety.

Kristin Neff highlights this beautifully when she says, "Continually feeding our need for positive self-evaluation is a bit like stuffing ourselves with candy. We get a brief sugar high, then a crash."

When our perfectionism is fed by achievement, we can increase our confidence by weaning ourselves off our perpetual performance. When we slowly reduce the things we're doing to be perfect, we discover that we don't have to be. And this makes it easier to choose sustainable, authentic living instead of the perfectionism anxiety spiral.

Further Reading

Mothers Are Made: How One Mom Overcame Perfectionism, Self-Doubt, Loneliness, and Anxiety and Became a Better and Happier Parent by Danielle Sherman-Lazar

Operating Instructions by Anne Lamott

The Gifts of Imperfection by Brené Brown

The Perfectionist's Guide to Losing Control: A Path to Peace and Power by Katherine Morgan Schafler

How to Deal with a Permissive Habit

"Love to kids is not: I'll give you whatever you want. It's: I'm here and I'm not going anywhere, no matter what you throw at me."

—ABBY WAMBACH, *We Can Do Hard Things*

People often think that a control habit and a permissive habit are on opposite sides of the spectrum. One habit is about grasping control, the other's about completely releasing it. In practice, yes, they are opposites, but they share the same core problem: both habits prioritize the mind of only one person in the relationship while ignoring the needs of the other.

In a control habit, it's the parent's mind that's prioritized. In a permissive habit, it is the child's. Neither habit prioritizes genuine connection or healthy development.

A permissive habit is a chronic pattern of indulgence in which we consistently allow our children to forgo limits, boundaries, and expectations because of our unmanaged anxiety (see page 21).

Most of the time, a permissive habit takes root either because it was modeled for us by our caregivers or because we had parents with control habits (see page 160) that were so pronounced that we felt unloved by them. We're worried that our children won't feel loved by us, so we constantly give them what they ask for, even when it's not what they truly need.

This looks like:

- Letting our children's emotional reactions to our expectations change or alter what we expect, even when it's detrimental to their health, safety, or growth
- Having very few limits or expectations to avoid conflict with our children
- Using money or gifts regularly to gain our children's approval or cooperation
- Feeling extreme guilt when we say no or set a limit
- Checking constantly for our children's approval of our decisions
- Putting our own social, emotional, or financial needs in peril to keep our children satisfied with our choices

How Does a Permissive Habit Affect Our Children?

When we habitually relinquish our boundaries and expectations to gain our children's approval, we compromise their growth. Because we're unsteady in ourselves we end up denying them the guidance and structure they need to feel secure in themselves and in their relationships with us. This gets in the way of the #1 gift of a secure parent, to show them that we can handle what they feel. We're showing them that we can't deal with their feelings. We want their negative feelings to go away, so we quickly release our expectations and boundaries to keep the emotions at bay.

While a child being raised by a parent with a control habit can't trust their parent to offer them *the nurture, understanding, and connection they need*, a child being raised by a parent with a permissive habit can't trust their parent with the *sturdiness, consistency, and guidance that they need.*

The anxiety (see page 21) that's at the core of a permissive habit has a profound impact on our children's ability to regulate themselves. When we constantly gratify their requests in order to avoid facing their emotional reactions to limits, they learn to rely on external gratification to feel regulated. This puts them at risk of developing a numbing habit (see page 208).

The other impact is that our children won't develop a sense of healthy cooperative boundaries. We've modeled a one-person-focused relationship, which can lead them to follow our lead and give themselves over to other people's wants and need. Or they'll see their needs as so central in relationships that they'll struggle to make room for others (they might develop narcissistic tendencies themselves!).

Let's Grow!

If we're caught in a permissive habit, we need to deal with our anxiety and develop confidence in ourselves (see How to Deal with a Self-Doubt Habit on page 246) and our decisions. Then our children can rely on us to provide the boundaries and expectations they need to help them develop and grow.

Consistency is incredibly comforting for our kids. We need to be soft enough to care for their hearts, but sturdy enough to stay rooted even when their emotional instability is shaking our branches.

Here's how we switch from a permissive habit to implementing confident boundaries and expectations.

Fences Can Be Sturdy Without Being Spiky

Our children need us to establish and maintain boundaries in their lives so they can feel safe and know what to expect. This doesn't mean we have to be harsh or hurtful to keep the fences up. We can be creative in how we communicate our expectations and boundaries, and have grace for our children when they're learning how to respect and cope with disappointments.

I struggle to hold boundaries when my kids are super tired or tender, or when I'm super tired or tender and can fall prey to letting my limits freefall. But I've noticed that when I do, holding the boundary is even harder for them the next time, triggering me to respond more harshly to their push back even though it was my fault the boundary slipped. So when I'm having a hard time holding a limit, I tell myself, "Hold it now a *little*, or you'll have to hold it *even more later*."

Repeat after me: *"My children need me to create expectations and structures in their lives to help them grow and learn. They may have feelings about this at first, but over time they'll be glad that I parented them with guidance and not permissiveness."*

Our Needs Need to Be in the Mix Too

Our children are in a relationship with us, which means they need to learn how to share the space with us, especially as they grow older. This is training for other relationships in their lives. They need to be able to collaborate and share space and power with whoever they're close to, and we're their first teachers for that reality.

This morning my son wanted to skip the bus and get a breakfast sandwich from the gas station. I have a small but important window when I can exercise on Wednesday mornings between my son's bus and my daughters' departure to school forty minutes later.

While part of me wanted to be the easy-going mom and alleviate my son's morning grump with a fun outing before school, I knew that I would regret not taking care of myself in a way that my brain and body needed.

While it was challenging to hold my boundary when he responded with frustration and pleading, I knew that by the end of the day, he would have moved on and would come home to a mom who was more regulated and available as a result of having taken care of my need to move this old bone bag.

Repeat after me: *"It's important that I take care of myself and my limits too so that my children learn how to be in a mutual relationship and not expect others to revolve only around their needs."*

It's Better to Be Clear than Cloudy

When we establish a guideline or limit for our children, it's best to consult with our peers and ourselves to clarify our decision before we share it with our children. If we're cloudy about what we think is best, we can lose our footing when our children have a negative response. It's far kinder to them and to us to be clear about what our expectations are before presenting them to our children and processing their responses.

I recently had to change my expectations around library books. I love library books. I love my kids reading them, and I love reading them together with my kids. I *do not love* frantically searching the house every week for due or overdue library books.

I reached out to my teacher/administrator bestie to find out what she thought about me putting down a hard and fast rule concerning my role in finding library books. She approved of my idea, and I made an official edict:

Library books have an official spot in our living room. If you read a library book, you put it back there. If you lose a library book, it's your responsibility to find it and to pay for it if you can't.

Now when my kids lose their books, I can offer compassion and understanding about their predicament, but I can hold back on the resentment and stress I felt when I was unintentionally agreeing to be responsible for finding their books.

Repeat after me: *"I'm the parent, and it's often my job to make decisions regardless of my children's approval or emotional responses. I can always adjust when I notice it's not working well or if new information comes to light. But I can trust my decisions even when they're not popular at this stage of my children's understanding."*

Trusty Tidbit

EXPERIENCE BUILDS CONFIDENCE

When our kids are pushing us (or "lawyering up" as I like to call it) to relax our expectations or boundaries, it is easy to get shaky on our structure or worry that we're being unkind or unreasonable.

When I'm feeling shaky over a limit I've set, I ask myself this question: "If I don't hold this expectation/limit/boundary, is there a life skill my child will miss out on learning now and therefore lose confidence over later?"

For example, if I'm asking my child to wait their turn somewhere and they lose their mind and another parent offers to let them go first, I likely decline the offer. Because learning to wait in line is an important skill that will increase social connections in my child's life.

I can stay compassionate and calm as I keep my child in their place in line, and I don't need to do this every single time, but I do the majority of the time. Our children will benefit greatly if we stay firm on scenarios that help them build skills such as patience, consideration of others, and delayed gratification. Even if they're pissed in the short term!

Compassionate Self-Talk Scripts

- *"Our children can't feel secure in their relationships with us if they can feel we're sacrificing our own well-being to appease them."*
- *"It's not my job to prevent my children from experiencing discomfort or pain; it is my job to prevent them from experiencing discomfort and pain in isolation."*
- *"If I can't do something for my children without building up resentment or feeling like a martyr, then I need to find a different solution for them to have their needs met so I can protect my relationship with them."*
- *"I don't have to work to be worthy of my children's love, I just have to work to accept that they won't always feel pleased with what I choose to do or not do for their well-being."*

Further Reading

Discipline Without Damage: How to Get Your Kids to Behave Without Messing Them Up by Vanessa Lapointe

Parenting Decolonized (podcast) with Yolanda Williams

Raising Securely Attached Kids by Eli Harwood

The Whole-Brain Child: Revolutionary Strategies to Nurture Your Child's Developing Mind by Daniel J. Siegel, MD, and Tina Payne Bryson, PhD

Tiny Humans, Big Emotions: How to Navigate Tantrums, Meltdowns, and Defiance to Raise Emotionally Intelligent Children by Alyssa Blask Campbell and Lauren Elizabeth Stauble

Very Intentional Parenting: Awakening the Empowered Parent Within by Destini Ann Davis

How to Deal with a

Self-Doubt Habit

"Always remember you are braver than you believe, stronger than you seem, and smarter than you think."

—**CHRISTOPHER ROBIN**, *Pooh's Grand Adventure*

We all doubt ourselves at times. Life is too messy and complex to *always* believe in ourselves and our perspectives, choices, and desires. Plus, having moments of self-doubt is essential to being a connected parent. Our children need us to have navigated self-doubt enough that we've gained the skills necessary to help them when it visits them.

But a self-doubt *habit* is another thing entirely. When we constantly or consistently doubt ourselves, we're not able to be sturdy and reliable for our children. If we don't trust ourselves, how can we expect them to trust us?

Signs of a Self-Doubt Habit

- Mostly or always crowd-sourcing decisions out of fear of messing up
- Rarely or never feeling confident in our choices or ideas
- Often second-guessing everything we do with a large helping of panic
- Frequent internal or external negative self-talk
- Quickly changing our minds when someone doesn't agree with us
- Regularly locking onto advice without first consulting our own feelings about an issue
- Frequently working overtime to be *liked* by other people instead of working to be *known*

Distorted Mirrors: The Roots of Self-Doubt

We all need positive relational mirrors in our lives, people who can accurately reflect our worthiness and capability back to us so we can believe in ourselves. When our early caregivers are accurate mirrors for us, they respond to our joy with delight, to our mistakes with support, and to our tenderness and emotions with calm empathy.

If our caregivers couldn't relate to us in those ways, the reflections we saw of ourselves were distorted, especially if our caregivers were cruel, critical, or overly harsh with us.

Without accurate mirroring from childhood caregivers, we were denied an essential ingredient for believing in ourselves. Chronic self-doubt is an internal model developed as a result of insecure attachment experiences in childhood. Human children need to know that they're seen, heard, understood, and validated in their internal experiences and external presence.

If we constantly question our perspectives, choices, and worthiness to belong, we should look back and acknowledge that our childhood experiences made it hard for us to trust ourselves and feel worthy.

Perhaps our caregivers couldn't give us the validation and confidence we needed because they were knee-deep in their own insecurities.

Or maybe they were overly critical or harsh with us because they had an ingrained control habit.

Perhaps our parents were so busy trying to launch our family out of poverty that they had little or no energy left to respond to our emotional needs.

Maybe our parents were so wounded that they were threatened by us and denied our capacity or worthiness in order to feel better about themselves.

Whatever the reason, we need to be honest with ourselves about the nature of those early relationships and how they impacted our self-confidence. Then we need to find people in our lives who can help us feel encouraged, validated, and understood, and then work to learn how to offer those same things to ourselves. We're editing our inner voices by changing the external voices we hold inside.

We don't get to decide what kind of caregiving we receive in childhood, but we do get to decide whether we hold onto the messages we received about ourselves as a result.

How Our Self-Doubt Habits Affect Our Children

When we chronically doubt ourselves, it makes it far harder for our children to trust in our reliability. If we're stuck in a pattern of denying our worthiness or second-guessing our desires or boundaries, our children can't rest in our presence or rely on us to offer them confidence in times when they feel wobbly or unsure.

This habit compromises our ability to give gift #1 to our children, to show them we can handle what they feel, because we're clearly struggling to handle what *we* feel. We haven't yet learned how to shut down shame gremlins (see page 129), and are instead entertaining them in our sense of ourselves.

It also compromises our ability to give them gift #5, to show them that we accept them for their full, authentic selves. Why? Because if we can't accept our full, authentic selves, it makes it much harder for them to trust that we can accept theirs. Even if we can.

Let's Grow!

The opposite of self-doubt is self-assurance. Feeling self-assured is, of course, easier said than done when we've spent many years questioning ourselves. Luckily there are things we can do to change the tides in our relationships with ourselves in the same way we can change the tides in any relationship we care about. The two most important aspects to work on are how we relate to ourselves and our decision-making processes.

Become Your Own BFF

One of the most profound ways we can deal with our self-doubt is to actively change the way that we relate to ourselves. This is such an important part of our growth and development that it's part of every single section of this book (I assume you've noticed this by now).

This happens in two ways: the way we treat our bodies and the way we talk to ourselves (in our heads and out loud).

If no one responded to your needs with nurture or spoke compassionately to you growing up, then making these changes might feel extra cheesy at first. You had to adapt to a world without close, compassionate responses, which means that you also had to tell yourself a story about not wanting or needing that type of care. This means you'll probably cringe now when some therapist in a book tells you to start treating yourself with compassion. That's to be expected, but please don't let it derail you. This is one of the most important things you can do for your children.

When we develop a habit of showing ourselves respect and care by speaking to ourselves with compassion, it changes us. We become calmer and more receptive in our presence, and less fragile, prickly, and defensive in our relationships with our children.

We're going to start by changing our self-talk because we tend to take better care of ourselves when we speak to ourselves with kindness.

Three forms of positive self-talk:

1 Affirmations: saying positive things to ourselves about who we are ("You're an incredibly caring human") and about what we do ("You work so hard and show up so fully").

2. Reassurance: responding to feelings of tenderness or insecurity with gentle care and understanding ("It makes sense you're feeling this way, but it's not true about who you are or what you're capable of").
3. Encouragement: reminding ourselves that we're capable of doing things, even when we're worried or uncertain, is a beautiful way to decrease self-doubt. I always refer to myself with my maiden last name when I'm doing this, a side effect of being an athlete in my youth I suppose ("You've got this, Fehler, knock it down, girl!").

If you struggle to find sentences to say to yourself in any of these areas, ask someone you know to write up some sentences they feel toward you for affirmation, reassurance, or encouragement, and start saying those things to yourself to help you get started.

Practicing Self-Care

The more we treat ourselves with kindness and care, the more we trust ourselves. Self-doubt is, in essence, a lack of trust in ourselves, so when we become our own personal trustworthy caretakers, it becomes much easier to kick a self-doubt habit and replace it with a self-trust habit.

Start with the small stuff and work your way up:

- Brushing your teeth, taking showers, etc.
- Getting ample rest, nutrition, and sunlight
- Moving your body in ways that help you feel strong and alive
- Filling your mind with things that give you hope and inspiration (hopefully reading this book is already doing that for you, but also great art, film, novels, nature, etc.)
- Letting go of people who don't treat you well

- Making a budget for financial well-being
- Creating art in whatever form suits your fancy

The steps you take to show your body and soul that you matter to you will help you be a better ally to yourself and clearer on what you feel, need, and want. All things that will make it easier to give your children the five gifts of a secure parent.

Decision Precision

One of the painful parts of being in a self-doubt habit is the constant feeling of indecision. And if you've struggled to trust yourself, I'm guessing you struggle to understand how other people seem to make decisions quickly and with little emotional fanfare. Let's dig into how to make a confident decision when you've spent years in decision paralysis.

I find it relevant that the prefix of the word "decide" means "to cut off." The process of choosing something always involves *not choosing* something else. Whether we have strong self-trust or we struggle with self-doubt, decisions, especially big ones, involve a fair amount of loss.

I share this because I think self-assurance can feel impossible to grasp when you've been shrouded in a cloud of self-doubt for a long time. The expectation is that when you stop doubting yourself, you'll feel completely confident in your choices without any uncertainty or doubt. But the reality is that no one gets to know the future before they make a decision. We learn about the impact of our choices in hindsight, not foresight.

If you've spent years in a self-doubt spiral, healing will look like making choices *even though they might be wrong or lead to negative outcomes,* not knowing for certain that all the choices you make are right. The goal is to learn how to make choices that *feel right for you* and let fate handle the rest. Sometimes the things you choose will be fantastic, and other times they'll bite you in the butt.

Finding out what choice feels right for you is about being clear on who you are and what you're about. For instance, if you see yourself as someone who cares about making the world a more connected place, then you should consider your choices based on that identity and your goals within it. When you're faced with whether to end a friendship, consider whether you feel connected and able to offer care within the relationship, or if you feel emotionally disconnected and distant. Say yes to the first answer and no to the second.

If you're asked to join a committee for the local sewage group, make sure your passion lies in waste management. If not it's okay that you're not interested. Sure you might regret saying no later on if you find out that you could have helped to stop a major toxic spill later that year, but it doesn't mean you made the wrong choice. It just means that something bad happened that you had no control over.

Compassionate hindsight is also a part of being self-assured. Being able to look back at a decision we made, understand why we made that decision, and honor that it was our best choice at the time. We're much more likely to learn and grow from our past mistakes if we can look at them with compassion.

Trusty Tidbit

IS IT TRULY SELF-DOUBT? OR DOUBT THAT OTHERS CAN HANDLE OUR CONFIDENCE WITHOUT RETALIATION?

So many of us have learned painfully that our talents, capacity, lovability, sparkle, and shine are threats to the deeply insecure people in our lives. This "lesson" is especially disorienting when the people we learn it from are attachment figures in our lives, including our parents, siblings, friends, and sweethearts.

We might not be struggling with self-doubt but with finding people who can handle our self-assurance.

Self-doubt can be a masking strategy that keeps us looking less threatening to people with narcissistic wounds. When important people in our lives feel threatened by our freedom or confidence, we forgo those precious gifts to preserve the relationships and avoid retribution.

When we're raising our children, it's our job to reclaim our self-alliance and let go of relationships that require us to shrink ourselves. If we don't our children will learn to shrink themselves too. Self-doubt is learned and inherited, not innate.

If people dislike your health, success, clear vision, ability to be silly and fun, capacity to build relationships, generosity, creativity, or whatever other jewels you possess, remember that the problem isn't your sunshine; it's their sensitivity to the sun.

Shine on.

Compassionate Self-Talk Scripts

- *"It's sad that no one was able to help me feel confident in myself as a child, but it doesn't mean I'm not capable of learning how to feel confident in myself now."*
- *"It's not possible to know the future, but I can learn to know myself and make my best guesses by listening closely when I am faced with a decision."*
- *"Just because someone disagrees with me doesn't mean they're right about what I feel or need."*
- *"I'm the greatest expert on myself and can trust myself when something feels right or wrong, regardless of what other people think."*

Further Reading

How to Be Yourself: Quiet Your Inner Critic and Rise Above Social Anxiety by Ellen Hendriksen
Own Your Greatness by Dr. Lisa Orbé-Austin and Dr. Richard Orbé-Austin
Securely Attached: Transform Your Attachment Patterns into Loving, Lasting Romantic Relationships by Eli Harwood
The Gifts of Imperfection by Brené Brown
The Impostor Phenomenon by Pauline Rose Clance
The Secret Thoughts of Successful Women by Valerie Young

The Deal with Dealing Onward

I'm so thankful that you joined me in this uphill hike of learning how to avoid the goombas that get in the way of our relationships with our children. That was no small feat. I'm sorry if you got blisters or lost a toenail along the way.

I hope the breathtaking sight of a deeply positive relationship with your offspring came into view and gave you the inspiration you needed to become a regular hiker. And most importantly, I hope you gained more compassion toward yourself.

Because of course our quest is ongoing; we're not finished after working on ourselves for a bit. We continue to face new mountains and obstacles. Sometimes we even get lost and have to go back and rescale a mountain we've already climbed. But we keep going. Not only for our children but also for ourselves.

As you journey onward, working to give your children the five gifts of a secure relationship with you (page x), I want to leave you with five gifts from me to take with you on your trip:

1. You are capable of emotional growth and repair. It's already in your DNA.
2. You are worthy of the peace, confidence, and connection that come from emotional growth.
3. Your emotional growth will have ripples that reach far beyond you and your children.
4. You will continue to falter, fall, and flop at times. So will I. It's part of the hike.
5. You are making the world a safer and more connected place for all of us by changing the things you can and taking responsibility for whatever sh*t you need to deal with.

Love on.

Appendices

How to Write an

"I Wish I Had Known" Letter

After reading through this book, you're probably now aware of a thing or two that you wish you'd done differently in your parenting journey. If your kids are itty-bitty, you only need to work on growing and healing whatever issue you recognize needs your attention. But if your children are old enough to process an apology, this letter is a template to help you express genuine remorse for the things you didn't know before.

And no, it's never too late to make amends for our actions or inactions. It doesn't mean our children will automatically embrace and forgive us, but it will be an opportunity for them to heal on a deeper level, and that's a gift every parent can offer, no matter how late. Your kids might be thirteen or thirty-two, either way, there's power in acknowledging that you see your earlier missteps.

To my daughter/son/child/lovebug/darling,

I've been reflecting on our relationship, and I've realized there are some things I've done (or not done) that hurt you. I'm writing this letter to acknowledge some of the mistakes I realize I've made and to try to apologize to you for them.

You don't need to talk about this with me if you're not ready to. Nor do you need to feel a certain way. I understand that just saying sorry doesn't automatically make something right. Take whatever time you need to process this and care for yourself in whatever way feels right. This is not about me, it's about how I hurt you. I hope that hearing my words about these things will validate some of what you've experienced with me and help you to feel understood in ways you haven't before. I also hope it will help you heal any way you need to.

If I had a do-over, I would do

__________________ *instead of* __________________

__________________ *instead of* __________________

__________________ *instead of* __________________

I'm so sorry that I did not hear you when you said _______________ *to me. I wish I'd listened more deeply and had a different response.*

If there are other things I haven't acknowledged here that are still hurting you that you want me to understand, I'm here to listen. I'll take in whatever you say and work through it so I can continue to grow and you can continue to share honestly with me whenever you feel hurt by me, either from past mistakes or present flubs.

Nothing in the world matters more to me than you. I'm here to talk through anything you want and will keep working on myself so that hopefully you can rely on me more in the future.

Love,

I hope this letter brings you closer to healing both yourself and your relationship with your children in whatever small or big ways you need.

How to Respond When Your Child Gives You Critical Feedback

It is never easy when our children give us critical feedback. It can be painful when they're four years old and calling us "mean" or when they're twenty-two and letting us know that they don't feel we're doing our job to help address the climate crisis.

And it is always *hard, hard, hard* when they share with us about issues in our relationship or life that have hurt them deeply. Perhaps they tell us we've been unavailable when they needed us or that we were overly harsh or anxious in a way that made it hard for them to rely on us fully. That type of feedback is quintessentially hard to hear. But they need us to hear it. So here are some tips to help the process.

Remember that "critical" means two different things: it can mean *cruel or harsh*, or it can mean *important*. When our children come to us with critical feedback, it's essential that we interpret their "critical" as important. We should be careful not to get defensive about potential anger or any harsh interpretations that the information may come wrapped up in.

Why? Because when our children come to us with feedback, they're making efforts to tell us what they need from us. Even if they tell us we've failed at something, what we do in response to their important information is vital for us to repair and move forward.

When your child gives you negative feedback, remember:

1. Your first goal is to listen and truly understand. No defending, explaining, or deflecting. Just hearing.
2. Your second goal is to feel empathetic toward your child. To let yourself catch their emotions and truly connect to what they're feeling.
3. Your third goal is to communicate heartbreak on their behalf (My heart is breaking to know that you've been feeling this way. Not *you're breaking my heart* by feeling this way). Demonstrate your care by showing them you can stay with their feelings without flooding them with your own.
4. Take notes for future engagements. Ask them what they need to feel good moving forward in your relationship.

If we're able to stay open and caring when our children offer critical feedback, it makes it easier for them to trust us and work on bringing future feedback with less defensiveness.

How to Get Your Partner to Read Something

One of the hardest parts of learning and growing is being in close relationships with people who are not yet interested in the path we've started. Especially when that person is your partner in raising your children.

There's no way to guarantee that our sweethearts or co-parents will join us in a connection-focused cycle-breaking journey as parents. But that doesn't mean we can't try to invite them to the emotional growth party. It does mean, however, that we need to be intentional in how we do it.

Here are a few tips to help you effectively ask someone to read a topic or two from this book (or any other growth-focused book you think they should read).

1. **Don't Let Panic Lead the Conversation:** This is a process, not a rescue. When we approach someone with panic energy, we'll almost undoubtedly be met with defensiveness. The energy we bring can get in the way of the message. Offer without pressure.

2. **Listen Before You Leap:** Take the time to understand what the other person is thinking about these topics or your child's development. Listen for the wisdom they already possess to help cultivate trust in your relationship with them.
3. **Establish Mutuality:** Whether you like it or not, this is a person you had children with or are currently raising them with. Make sure you communicate that you see them as a partner and that you don't assume the leadership position on the topic. You're doing this together.
4. **Invitations over Interventions:** It tends to backfire when we push or prod people into doing self-work. Make sure your energy feels more like you're sharing a food you love than shaming them or condescending about the food they're currently eating.
5. **Pack the Proof in the Pudding:** The more you do this work, the more your people will see how it has changed you and your relationship with your children. Focus on the mess on your side of the street, and other people will feel far more enthusiastic about learning what you know.
6. **Put Care at the Center:** If you're asking your person to read something, make sure the message is, "I adore you so much and I know how much you've been struggling to feel *x*, *y*, *z*, and I think this might be something that could help. I could be wrong, of course, but I can't help wanting to get you relief; you deserve to feel all the way good in this arena."

When you're trying to win someone over to a practice of secure relating, remember that many experiences molded them into their current patterns. It will take time to unpeel that onion and get to the core of their heart. Give them as much grace, time, and acceptance as you can muster. Understanding them with compassion will have the most effect on them moving forward.

Sample Script:

"I know that reading books about parenting and self-growth is more my thing than yours, but it would mean the world to me if you would read a few things in this book. I found myself thinking about what you've been through and what I know matters to you, and I think that a few of these things will be meaningful for you to feel more confident/more connected/ easier on yourself. I'd also be more than happy to read anything you want me to if you have something similar in mind for me."

How to

Get Yourself to Go to Therapy

(and Find a Good Therapist)

Going to therapy is inherently vulnerable, which means that starting therapy usually comes with some anticipatory nerves. It takes a leap of faith to enter a room with a person who doesn't know us from Adam and then proceed to open up to them about our incredibly complex lives.

And we all know therapy is likely to involve tears and some revelations that we may have been denying. And if we don't have a personal history of people responding empathetically to our tears, the discomfort with therapy ratchets upward.

But there's a difference between being nervous, or even scared, that therapy might come with some growing pains and being so terrified of it that we never even try.

Some common reasons why we might stall out on or resist going to therapy:

- We imagine that all we'll discover in therapy is that we're bad people or more broken than we thought.
- We assume that the process will bring only pain and not growth or hope.
- We cling to every bad possible story that we hear about therapists or therapy and ignore the many more people who have been helped by it.
- We make excuses for why we can't go at this moment in time and always kick the can down the road.

Before I try to convince you to work through this fear and find a good therapist who can support your growth journey, I want to be straight about a few things.

Not All Therapy Is Effective or Good

Why? Because not every therapist and client are the right fit for each other.

Why? It could be cultural differences, a personality mismatch, a treatment approach mismatch, or bad timing.

Some Therapy Is Straight Up Bad

Why? A therapist lacks necessary training in the issue you're navigating and is practicing out of their scope of competence (bad advice), a therapist is unethical and relationally corrupt in some way (abusive), or a therapist lacks the level of empathy and care that the work requires (emotionally inept or neglectful).

But Good and Effective Therapy Is Life-Changing

Why? Because when we're met face-to-face with a human being who has the capacity to see us clearly, hear us fully, and help us thoroughly, we can make changes in our behaviors, thoughts, emotional states, and relational patterns that we could never make without that level of care and support from someone else.

Which is why we pay therapists (or our insurance or social services do). Because in no other relationship would it be okay for us to take up all the attention and space, and to continue to do dumb sh*t and still be welcomed back to keep trying. Therapists are compensated financially so that we can take up all the space we need to heal and grow.

Think of Finding a Therapist as a Dating Process

You wouldn't expect yourself to find "the one" after only one internet search or initial meet-up, right? The same goes for therapy. Give yourself a chance to find someone who's a good fit for you.

1. Ask friends for suggestions and ask them to ask their friends too if you want to keep a little more distance between your therapist and your community (recommended).
2. Consider what aspects of cultural competency are essential that your therapist understands about you/your culture, and be prepared to ask about how they offer support/varied approaches based on your challenges.
3. Ask therapists for an initial free fifteen-to-twenty-minute phone consultation (most will do that for you because they also want to avoid a bad-fit relationship).

4. Listen to your gut on whether you felt the person connected to you, was confident in helping you, and offered you some hope or relief in that initial conversation.
5. If you have a good initial connection, give it four to five sessions and see how it goes. If, after that, you don't find the work helpful, cut bait and look for another option.
6. If the fit is right, you'll feel seen, cared for, challenged, and supported in meeting your goals, and you'll develop and grow demonstrably in that space.
7. It's okay if it's not a long-term relationship or if you outgrow a therapist over time. Sometimes what we need in a specific season makes a therapist a great fit, but then over time, we need someone/something different. That's growth! You don't owe a therapist anything other than the fee you pay for each session (oh and any sessions that you cancel last minute, if they have that policy!).

Resources

General

For therapists searchable by those offering sliding scale rates: Therapist.com | *Therapist.com*

For general, affordable healthcare services, including mental health services: National Association of Free and Charitable Clinics | *NAFCClinics.org*

A nonprofit network of mental health professionals offering low-cost care: Open Path Psychotherapy Collective | *OpenPathCollective.org*

For substance abuse treatment resources: Substance Abuse and Mental Health Services Administration | *SAMHSA.gov*

Specific Communities

For current/former foster youth (or anyone who has *ever* been system involved!): A Home Within | *AHomeWithin.org*

For low-cost psychotherapy available to the Asian community, see the Lotus Therapy Fund: Asian Mental Health Collective | *AsianMHC.org*

For Black women, girls, and nonbinary folks: Loveland Therapy Fund | TheLovelandFoundation.org

For free therapy available to the BIPOC community: BIPOC Therapy Fund | *MentalHealthLiberation.org*

For free therapy available to the queer community: National Queer & Trans Therapists of Color Network's Mental Health Fund | *NQTTCN.com*

For resources around Native American healthcare, including behavioral health: Indian Health Services, Map of Care | *IHS.gov*

Other Search Ideas

Ask your local Catholic charity organization, as they will offer low-cost/no-cost therapy services.

Check out your local university's counseling centers—often they offer free/low-cost services to students.

Make enquiries with your employer, as many offer Employment Assistant Program (EAP) therapy benefits that employees don't even know about!

Acknowledgments

To my sweetheart, Trevor, and to my three incredible children for understanding that my heart and brain are full of chatter that needs to be organized onto pages. Thank you for being proud of me and cheering me on as I continue to put my passion out into the world. You are my *why* and the best part of my life.

To all of my parents (bio and bonus) who have lived through decades of me studying an incredibly tender, albeit hopeful, topic. I'm incredibly lucky to have so many parents who love me.

To Amanda Fuenzalida for constantly fielding my brainstorms and always reading my drafts as soon as I mention them, and then for telling me that what I wrote was worth writing, even when I feel like a lost, nutty professor.

To my brother Scott for reminding me that there's always hope, and that what seems like the end of a sentence may actually be an incredibly redemptive semicolon waiting for a whole new idea.

To Skye Goodman, thank you for being the most incredible research assistant, business support, and heart family. You're always clear on what matters and thinking of every possible way we can work to support everyone on earth.

To Diana Cherry for your invaluable feedback and contributions to this manuscript, and for being an incredibly wise and kind friend. I'm so thankful for how you helped me to consider all the unique humans who will experience this book.

To my editor Jill Saginario, I literally cannot imagine a book without your support and insight. Thank you for being so willing to jump into these depths with me, and for telling me when I've turned up the cheese too high or forgotten to put enough of myself into the text. You're simply incredible, and your friendship has been a massive bonus to this book-making journey.

To the Still Got It Gals for always standing by my side and listening to me process and vent when I'm in the thick of my growth areas. And for being people who are constantly learning and growing yourselves.

To Meggo Shahabi, Whitney Losee, Abby Wong, Heather Baker, Sarah Dutcher, Matt Herz, Kelley Gray, Jon Fogel, Welles and Jeremy Bricker, Catherine Jensen, Shauna Gauthier, Callie Moore, Kaylyn Wilson, Maggie Nick, Alyssa Blask-Campbell, Kristin Galant, and Maria Guerra for being cheerleaders and companions on this wild ride.

To Janelle and all of our PASS Center therapists and Attachment Labs coaches who have shared stories and given suggestions to help this book become a reality.

To all my incredible clients who have trusted me with your heartache, your hopes, and your desire to grow and change. You live inside my heart in a sacred space, and so many of the things we've uncovered together are alive inside this book.

To my incredible book team, Ashley Hong, Brenna Licalzi, Peggy Gannon, Anna Goldstein, Rachel Sims, María Jesús Aguilo, Lindsay Wilkes-Edrington, all the staff at Blue Star Press and Sasquatch Books, and the incredible artists Maricor/Maricar. Your work on this project has been invaluable to me.

To everyone who follows me on the internet on Instagram, Facebook, or Tiktok @attachmentnerd or has been a part of the Attachment Nerd Herd, your presence has a massive impact on my life and on these messages reaching all the people who need them. You are a gift in my life, and I am so glad you are here.

Notes

Introduction

x “It’s a quest that has been journeyed by many courageous parents, and it has been validated as a worthy cause in the rich body of research on the parent-child relationship over the past century, or close to it.” Diane Benoit and Kevin C. H. Parker, “Stability and Transmission of Attachment across Three Generations,” *Child Development* 65, no. 5 (1994): 1444–1456, https://doi.org/10.1111/j.1467-8624.1994.tb00828.x.

x “It’s a quest that has been journeyed by many courageous parents, and it has been validated as a worthy cause in the rich body of research on the parent-child relationship over the past century, or close to it.” Mona D. Fishbane, “Healing Intergenerational Wounds: An Integrative Relational–Neurobiological Approach,” *Family Process* 58, no. 4 (2019): 796–818, https://doi.org/10.1111/famp.12488.

x “It’s a quest that has been journeyed by many courageous parents, and it has been validated as a worthy cause in the rich body of research on the parent-child relationship over the past century, or close to it.” John Bowlby, *A Secure Base: Clinical Applications of Attachment Theory.* (Routledge, 1988), 118–156.

The Feelings

3 “Teaching our children that it is okay to feel and that we will be there to support them is the path toward helping them develop confidence, empathy, and resilience.” Elizabeth D. Krause, Tamar Mendelson, and Thomas R. Lynch, “Childhood emotional invalidation and adult psychological distress: the mediating role of emotional inhibition,” *Child Abuse & Neglect* 27, no. 2 (2003): 199–213, https://doi.org/10.1016/S0145-2134(02)00536-7.

How to Deal with Feeling ANGRY

13 “Anger can become a problem in our lives and our children’s lives if we don’t know how to manage our responses to it.” K. Renk, V. Phares, and J. Epps, “The relationship between parental anger and behavior problems in children and adolescents,” *Journal of Family Psychology* 13, no. 2 (1999): 209–227, https://doi.org/10.1037/0893-3200.13.2.209.

17 "When we accurately tell ourselves we are experiencing an emotion, it helps to calm the cortical firing in our brains." Daniel J Siegel and Tina Payne Bryson, *The Whole-Brain Child Workbook: Practical Exercises, Worksheets and Activities to Nurture Developing Minds* (PESI Publishing & Media, 2015), 26-34.

18 "Anger is a secondary emotion." Brené Brown, *Atlas of the Heart: Mapping Meaningful Connection and the Language of Human Experience* (Random House, 2021), 218-238.

How to Deal with Feeling ANXIOUS

21 "Anxiety is a specialized form of fear." Cornelius T. Gross and Newton S. Canteras, "The many paths to fear," *Nature Reviews Neuroscience* 13 (2012): 651–658, https://doi.org/10.1038/nrn3301.

24 "Anxiety is not a trait or a permanent condition; it's an emotional state, and with effort, can be reduced to levels that are helpful instead of harmful." Peter J. Lang, "The Cognitive Psychophysiology of Emotion: Fear and Anxiety," in *Anxiety and the Anxiety Disorders*, ed. A. H. Tuma, and J. Maser (Routledge, 1985), 131–170. https://doi.org/10.4324/9780203728215-10.

26 "Caffeine can have a serious effect on our anxiety states." D. M. Veleber and D. I. Templer, "Effects of caffeine on anxiety and depression," *Journal of Abnormal Psychology* 93, no. 1 (1984): 120–122, https://doi.org/10.1037/0021-843X.93.1.120.

26 "Alcohol acts as a depressant in our nervous systems." H. E. Himwich, "The Physiology of Alcohol," *JAMA* 163, no. 7 (1957): 545–549, https://doi.org/10.1001/jama.1957.82970420003009.

How to Deal with Feeling BODY DISGUST

40 "Disgust always stems from things we have learned in our social worlds." Marie-Claude Paquette and Kim Raine, "Sociocultural context of women's body image," *Social Science & Medicine* 59, no. 5 (2004): 1047–1058, https://doi.org/10.1016/j.socscimed.2003.12.016.

40 "Disgust always stems from things we have learned in our social worlds." Alyson K. Spurgas, "Body Image and Cultural Background," *Sociological Inquiry* 75, no. 3 (2005): 297–316, https://doi.org/10.1111/j.1475-682X.2005.00124.

How to Deal with Feeling JEALOUS OF OUR CHILDREN

64 "Narcissism is a profound pattern of self-centered mentality and behavior with a profound absence of attention or attunement to others unless for self-gratification." Stephen K. Huprich, "Malignant self-regard: A

self-structure enhancing the understanding of masochistic, depressive, and vulnerable narcissistic personalities," *Harvard Review of Psychiatry* 22, no. 5 (2014): 295–305, https://doi.org/10.1097/HRP.0000000000000019.

How to Deal with Feeling JUDGED

70 "A side effect of growth is losing people who liked you better when you were without boundaries or engaged in behavior similar to theirs." @ nedratawwab. Instagram.com, accessed July 2, 2025, www.instagram.com/p/DF3hZnQvYmt/?hl=en.

How to Deal with Feeling LONELY

81 "Togetherness in our relationships positively impacts our longevity and well-being." Antigoni Mertika, Paschalia Mitskidou, and Anastassios Stalikas, "'Positive Relationships" and their impact on wellbeing: A review of current literature,' *Psychology: The Journal of the Hellenic Psychological Society* 25, no. 1 (2020): 115–127, https://doi.org/10.12681/psy_hps.25340.

How to Deal with Feeling POWERLESS

275 "Our internal models of the world are profoundly influential on our children." Judith A. Crowell and S. Shirley Feldman, "Mothers' Internal Models of Relationships and Children's Behavioral and Developmental Status: A Study of Mother-Child Interaction," *Child Development* 59, no. 5 (1988): 1273–1285, https://doi.org/10.2307/1130490.

275 "Our internal models of the world are profoundly influential on our children." Jenny Macfie, Nancy L. Mcelwain, Renate M. Houts, and Martha J. Cox, "Intergenerational transmission of role reversal between parent and child: Dyadic and family systems internal working models." *Attachment & Human Development* 7, no. 1 (2005): 51–65, https://doi.org/10.1080/14616730500039663.

89 "Everything can be taken from a man but one thing: the last of the human freedoms—to choose one's attitude in any given set of circumstances, to choose one's own way." Viktor E. Frankl, *Man's Search for Meaning* (Beacon Press, 1992, 4th edition), 62.

91 Sabrina Felson, "What Is Box Breathing?" WebMD, effective April 27, 2025, accessed May 20, 2025, https://www.webmd.com/balance/what-is-box-breathing.

How to Deal with Feeling SHAME

132 "The more we share our shame with others, the less we feel it, and the less power it has over us." Daniel Fessler, "Shame in Two Cultures: Implications for Evolutionary Approaches," *Journal of Cognition and Culture* 4, no. 2 (2004): 207-262, https://doi.org/10.1163/1568537041725097.

How to Deal with Feeling STRESSED

135 "When we live in a chronic or intense state of stress response, we're no doubt exposing our children to increased stress." Ross A. Thompson, "Stress and Child Development," *The Future of Children* 24, no. 1 (2014): 41–59, http://www.jstor.org/stable/23723382.

138 "When we take a mindful moment to pay attention to physical tension, it helps our brains to release it. It signals to us that we're safe enough to stop and observe." Alessandro Grecucci, Edoardo Pappaianni, Roma Siugzdaite, Anthony Theuninck, and Remo Job, "Mindful Emotion Regulation: Exploring the Neurocognitive Mechanisms behind Mindfulness," *BioMed Research International* 2015, no. 1 (2015): 1–9, https://doi.org/10.1155/2015/670724.

How to Deal with Feeling TRAUMATIZED

148 "Complex trauma is often covert or confusing, making it harder to recognize, understand, and verbalize, making the narrative part of the trauma far more convoluted and trickier to edit." Pete Walker, *Complex PTSD: From Surviving to Thriving* (CreateSpace Independent Publishing Platform, 2013), 40-45.

How to Deal with a BIAS HABIT

167 "Children have never been very good at listening to their elders, but they have never failed to imitate them." James Baldwin, *Nobody Knows My Name: More Notes of a Native Son* (Dial Press 1961), 173.

168 "Bias is a natural inclination for or against an idea, object, group, or individual." "Defining Bias," University of Chicago, accessed May 20, 2025, https://help.uchicago.edu/bias-education-and-support-team/bias/.

169 "Someone caught up in bigotry is a person who hates or refuses to accept the members of a particular group (such as a racial or religious group)." *The Britannica Dictionary*, www.britannica.com/dictionary/bigot.

169 "We all have biases and our biases are often unconsciously driving our choices." A. G. Greenwald, B. A. Nosek, and M. R. Banaji, "Understanding and using the implicit association test: I. An improved scoring algorithm," *Journal of Personality and Social Psychology* 85, no. 2 (2003): 197.

169 "It's common for us to be unfair to our fellow human beings accidentally." C. Pritlove, C. Juando-Prats, K. Ala-Leppilampi, and J. A. Parsons, "The good, the bad, and the ugly of implicit bias," *The Lancet* 393, No. 10171 (2019): 502-504.

171 "In the last year, 39 percent of LGBTQ youths have seriously considered suicide, including 46 percent of transgender and nonbinary youths." "2024 U.S. National Survey on the Mental Health of LGBTQ+ Young People," The Trevor Project, www.thetrevorproject.org/survey-2024/.

How to Deal with a BLAMING HABIT

179 "A blaming habit is damaging to our children's sense of security in their relationships with us." Rivka Yahav and Shiomo A. Sharlin, "Blame and family conflict: symptomatic children as scapegoats," *Child & Family Social Work* 7, no. 2 (2002): 91-98, https://doi.org/10.1046/j.1365-2206.2002.00231.x.

180 "The words "responsibility" and "accountability" share the same suffix "ability," which refers to the ability to do something." *Oxford Advanced Learner's Dictionary,* Oxford University Press, www.oxfordlearnersdictionaries.com/us/definition/american_english/able-ible#able-ible__39.

180 "The prefix of "responsibility" is "response" or "respond" meaning to answer." *Oxford Advanced Learner's Dictionary,* Oxford University Press, www.oxfordlearnersdictionaries.com/us/definition/english/respond.

How to Deal with a DISTRACTION HABIT

200 "Attention deficit hyperactivity disorder is a real neurological condition that can affect our ability to implement these practices for protecting presence." Mikka Nielsen, "ADHD and Temporality: A Desynchronized Way of Being in the World," *Medical Anthropology* 36, no. 3 (2017): 260–272, https://doi.org/10.1080/01459740.2016.1274750.

How to Deal with a PEOPLE-PLEASING HABIT

225 "A synonym for people-pleasing is fawning." Pete Walker, *Complex PTSD: From surviving to thriving* (CreateSpace, 2013), 40-45.

229 "A brave group of friends introduced me to the power and control wheel." "Understanding the Power and Control Wheel," https://www.theduluthmodel.org/wheels/understanding-power-control-wheel/.

How to Deal with a PERFECTIONISM HABIT

233 "Perfectionism also increases the chance that our children will hide their reality from us when life inevitably gets messy." M. D. Marc H. Hollender, "Perfectionism," *Comprehensive Psychiatry* 6, no. 2 (1965): 94–103, https://doi.org/10.1016/S0010-440X(65)80016-5.

235 "Parents who can cultivate secure relationships are not remotely close to 100 percent." M. J. Bakermans-Kranenburg, M. H. van IJzendoorn, and F. Juffer, "Less is more: Meta-analyses of sensitivity and attachment interventions in early childhood," *Psychological Bulletin* 129, no. 2 (2003): 195–215, https://doi-org.libproxy1.usc.edu/10.1037/0033-2909.129.2.195.

235 "Secure parents are positively connected with children around 30-50 percent of the time." Susan S. Woodhouse, Julie R. Scott, Allison D. Hepworth, and Jude Cassidy, "Secure Base Provision: A New Approach to Examining Links Between Maternal Caregiving and Infant Attachment," *Child Development* 91, no. 1 (2020): e249—e265, https://doi.org/10.1111/cdev.13224.

237 "We can only turn up our sense of worthiness by being vulnerable and authentic with the safe and loving people in our lives." Michelle A. Harris and Ulrich Orth, "The link between self-esteem and social relationships: A meta-analysis of longitudinal studies," *Journal of Personality and Social Psychology* 119, no. 6 (2020): 1459–1477, https://doi.org/10.1037/pspp0000265.

How to Deal with a SELF-DOUBT HABIT

247 "Chronic self-doubt is an internal model developed as a result of insecure attachment experiences in childhood." Fei Shen, Yanhong Liu, and Mansi Brat, "Attachment, Self-Esteem, and Psychological Distress: A Multiple-Mediator Model," *The Professional Counselor* 11, no. 2 (2021): 129–142, https://doi.org/10.15241/fs.11.2.129.

252 "The prefix of the word "decide" means "to cut off." "Etymonline," https://www.etymonline.com/word/decide.

Index

C

D

E

F

G

H

T

U

V

W

Y

About the Author

ELI HARWOOD is a licensed therapist who lives in Colorado with her husband, Trevor, their three children, two cats, and five chickens. Eli has been nerding out on attachment research for the past two decades and is on a mission to help make the world a better place, one relationship at a time. She continues this mission in her clinical work, in her writing, and on social media, where she runs her mouth about attachment.

When she isn't working to make the world a more secure place, she's baking, cooking, playing dress-up with her kids, and organizing her embarrassingly large collection of dangly earrings.

Visit her at AttachmentNerd.com, or you can follow her on Instagram, Facebook, and YouTube (@attachmentnerd). For more help from Eli, head to AttachmentNerd.com to learn about coaching options, as well as virtual and in-person offerings of her Secure Parent Program. (For the virtual program, there is a "pay what you can" option available. Because every parent on earth truly deserves to have access to this information and support.)

For more resources and opportunities to learn from and connect with Eli scan this code!